Ellen N. La Motte

MANCHESTER
1824

Manchester University Press

Nursing History and Humanities

Series editors: Christine E. Hallett and Jane E. Schultz

This series provides an outlet for the publication of rigorous academic texts in the two closely related disciplines of Nursing History and Nursing Humanities, drawing upon both the intellectual rigour of the humanities and the practice-based, real-world emphasis of clinical and professional nursing.

At the intersection of Medical History, Women's History and Social History, Nursing History remains a thriving and dynamic area of study with its own claims to disciplinary distinction. The broader discipline of Medical Humanities is of rapidly growing significance within academia globally, and this series aims to encourage strong scholarship in the burgeoning area of Nursing Humanities more generally.

Such developments are timely, as the nursing profession expands and generates a stronger disciplinary axis. The MUP Nursing History and Humanities series provides a forum within which practitioners and humanists may offer new findings and insights. The international scope of the series is broad, embracing all historical periods and including both detailed empirical studies and wider perspectives on the cultures of nursing.

Previous titles in this series:

Mental health nursing: the working lives of paid carers in the nineteenth and twentieth centuries
Edited by Anne Borsay and Pamela Dale

Negotiating nursing: British Army sisters and soldiers in the Second World War
Jane Books

One hundred years of wartime nursing practices, 1854–1953
Edited by Jane Brooks and Christine E. Hallett

'Curing queers': Mental nurses and their patients, 1935–74
Tommy Dickinson

Histories of nursing practice
Edited by Gerard M. Fealy, Christine E. Hallett and Susanne Malchau Dietz

Nurse writers of the Great War
Christine Hallett

Who cared for the carers? A history of the occupational health of nurses, 1880–1948
Debbie Palmer

Colonial caring: A history of colonial and post-colonial nursing
Edited by Helen Sweet and Sue Hawkins

ELLEN N. LA MOTTE

NURSE, WRITER, ACTIVIST

LEA M. WILLIAMS

Manchester University Press

Published by Manchester University Press
Altrincham Street, Manchester M1 7JA, UK
www.manchesteruniversitypress.co.uk

British Library Cataloguing-in-Publication Data is available

ISBN 978 1 5261 2951 2 hardback

First published 2020

Typeset by Newgen Publishing UK

To Rob, Tess, and Zoe

Contents

Figures

Acknowledgements

I would like to thank the American Association for the History of Nursing for supporting my project with the H-15 Research Grant for 2014. The editors and readers of the organization's journal, *Nursing History Review*, especially Cynthia Connolly and Pat D'Antonio, were helpful and enthusiastic about my article, "Ellen N. La Motte: The Making of a Nurse, Writer, and Activist," published in 2015. The members of the AAHN provided useful and supportive feedback at the annual conferences about the ideas I was incubating and showed me the real value of collegiality. I thank Springer for permission to republish the article in parts of Chapters 1 and 2.

I extend my sincere thanks to the Office of Academic Research and the Faculty Development Program at Norwich University, through which I received an independent study leave to devote one semester to this project, several course releases, and a number of grants to conduct research and travel to conferences to present my work. Their assistance, along with the support of my deans and department chairs, enabled me to engage in the time-consuming research necessary for this book project.

Equally important to this project is the unflagging support I received from my third floor of Webb Hall comrades, Patricia Ferreira and Amy Woodbury Tease, who read parts of the manuscript and spent countless hours talking over the problems and questions that arose over the years of research and writing. Without that community, this project would have withered on the vine. Friends and colleagues also served as readers and I thank them for taking time out of their overloaded schedules to give my work their time and attention: Dan Lane, Kathleen McDonald, Sylvia Sievers (and her father Albert Sievers), and Jonathan Walters.

Others provided invaluable support as well, including the librarians at the Kreitzberg Library, Norwich University, who patiently responded to hundreds of ILL requests and answered various questions over the years. Librarians and archivists at many institutions also tracked down requests and sent me material; some extended particular kindness and generosity, including Lisa McCown, Special Collections and Archives, Washington and Lee Library, on one of my first major research trips. Students provided key assistance as well: Eric Weinhold read terrible microfilm; Joshua Chang Inman scanned hundreds of documents without which this book could not have been written, and Courtney Pileski worked on deciphering difficult-to-read primary documents.

I also wish to thank profoundly the La Motte family for inviting me into their home and allowing me access to hundreds of documents that provided the bedrock for this project. I cannot thank you enough for allowing me the privilege of studying these papers and incorporating them into my work.

I also owe thanks to Rob, Tess, and Zoe for letting me share our time and space with Ellen.

Abbreviations

AID	Alfred I. du Pont Papers, Washington and Lee University, Lexington, VA
AJN	*American Journal of Nursing*
CHM	Chicago History Museum
FMCP	Frederick Mortimer Clapp Papers, Yale Collection of American Literature, Beinecke Rare Book and Manuscript Library, Yale University, New Haven, CT
GSABTP	Gertrude Stein and Alice B. Toklas Papers, Yale Collection of American Literature, Beinecke Rare Book and Manuscript Library, Yale University, New Haven, CT
IDNA	Instructive District Nursing Association of Boston
IHIP	Inez Haynes Irwin Papers, Schlesinger Library, Radcliffe Institute, Harvard University, Cambridge, MA
IVNA	Baltimore Instructive Visiting Nurse Association
JBDP	Jesse Ball du Pont Papers, Washington and Lee University, Lexington, VA
JHMI	Alan Mason Chesney Medical Archives of the Johns Hopkins Medical Institutions, Baltimore, MD
JHNAM	*Johns Hopkins Nurses Alumnae Magazine*

JOL	*Journal of the Outdoor Life*
MBDS	Mary Bartlett Dixon Scrapbooks, Suffrage Collection, Sophia Smith Collection, Smith College, Northampton, MA
MDPC	Margaretta E. du Pont Coleman Papers, Hagley Museum and Library, Wilmington, DE
MP	Mencken Papers, Manuscripts and Archives Division, The New York Public Library
NARA	National Archives and Records Administration, Washington, DC
NAWSA	National American Woman Suffrage Association
SSCMD	Social Service Club of Maryland
SWGR	Society of Woman Geographers Records, Manuscript Division, Library of Congress, Washington, DC
TNA	The National Archives, Kew
WSPU	Women's Social and Political Union

Introduction: The making of a nurse, writer, and activist

In a 1951 alumni survey Ellen Newbold La Motte, a 1902 graduate of the Johns Hopkins Training School for Nurses, provided this succinct response to the request that she evaluate her impressions and experiences as a student nurse: "Nothing to evaluate. Did not like it."[1] In response to a second question, her assessment of her time as a graduate nurse was even terser: "Ditto."[2] By the time La Motte completed the survey she had long ago left nursing behind and had forged an independent life for herself during which she amassed myriad exceptional professional and personal experiences: in 1915 she waited out a zeppelin raid in a stairwell in Paris with Gertrude Stein and Picasso; she served as a nurse on the Western Front two years before the United States entered the war; the British Foreign Office suspected her of being a spy in 1916; she was a member of the Heterodoxy Club, a group of radical women who met in Greenwich Village; and in the 1930s she had tea at the White House with Eleanor Roosevelt and witnessed the coronation of Emperor Haile Selassie in Ethiopia. La Motte's curiosity and need for new intellectual challenges led to extremely diverse professional successes, driving her to build a career as a nurse, writer, and activist over three decades.

Her abilities as a writer advanced her career, enabling her to participate in local, regional, national, and international conversations with other professionals and casual readers about tuberculosis, women's suffrage, World War One, and the opium trade. Over the course of her life, she published seven books: *The Tuberculosis Nurse* (1914), a textbook for nurses, particularly those working with tuberculosis patients in large cities; *The Backwash of War* (1916), a collection of sketches about nursing on the Western Front in Belgium in 1915 and 1916;

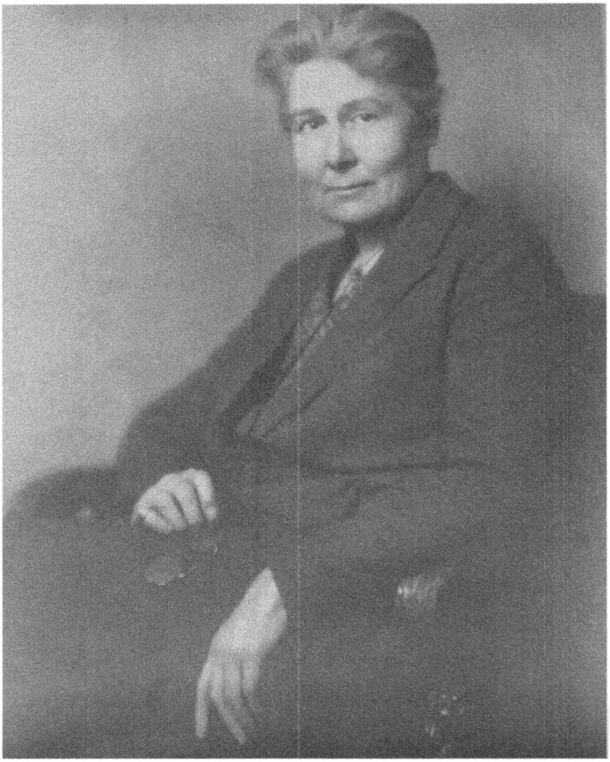

Figure 1 Portrait of La Motte, undated, probably 1920s

and five others that include short stories, narratives about her travels, and exposés of the devastating effects of the opium trade. She was also the author of many articles and stories published in newspapers, medical journals, publications dedicated to philanthropy and reform, and magazines with a broad national readership like the *Nation*, the *Century Magazine*, *Harper's*, and the *Atlantic Monthly*.

The range of these publications is a testament to the ever-changing interests La Motte nurtured during the first three decades of the twentieth century. While La Motte's claim that she liked nothing about her training and employment as a nurse rings true, an examination of the development of her working life reveals that nursing allowed her to hone her skills as a researcher, a writer, an executive, and an activist while engaging with crusades focused on public health issues and political rights for women. Like many women of her period La Motte found her way into the public eye through participation in "caring causes," shaping her professional self by speaking, writing, and advocating on behalf of others while using what she learned to build a career and an independent existence for herself. In 1928, thirty years after her initial application to Johns Hopkins, her nursing colleagues paid tribute to those three decades of research, writing, speaking, and service when she appeared on the cover of *Trained Nurse and Hospital Review*. They described her as a "world traveler, author, international authority on the opium traffic" who "made valued contributions" to "tremendous problems–social justice, health, war, opium."[3]

The article also says she was from "a family that had achieved widely in the arts" from whom she had "inherited broad vision and intuitive artistic feeling."[4] Scant information about the milieu in which she was raised, including whether it was creative or restrictive, is available although enough facts can be assembled to flesh out the bare bones of her life until she found her voice in 1901 and began her publishing career. Ellen Newbold La Motte was born in Louisville, Kentucky in 1873 and was brought up in Kentucky and Virginia by her parents, transplants from Pennsylvania and Delaware.[5] Her father, Ferdinand Lammot,[6] or Ferd as he was known to his family, grew up in a house plagued by illness and death, as many did in the mid-nineteenth century. His older brother, Allen, died of unidentified causes in 1845 at the age of two when Lammot was less than a year old.[7] His death was followed by that of Lammot's father, also named Ferdinand Fairfax Lammot, who died of "consumption" in 1849 at the age of forty, having struggled with the disease for five years.[8] His mother, Marietta Morse Allen, died of consumption a year and a half later at the age of thirty-seven. Lammot, and his sister, Margaretta Elizabeth La Motte, were orphaned by the time he was five and left to the care of his father's sister, Mary Augusta Lammot Hounsfield, in the Wilmington, Delaware area. Another aunt, Margaretta Elizabeth Lammot du Pont, had married Alfred V. du Pont in 1824. With the growing gunpowder business and other enterprises, the du Pont family was an important resource for Lammot as he sought career options outside Delaware. Lammot's grandfather, Daniel Lammot, father of Mary and Margaretta, was involved in manufacturing in southeastern Pennsylvania and was a business associate and friend of the du Ponts, indicating that the ties between the Lammots and du Ponts were long-standing.[9] Lammot took advantage of those ties, and in fall 1865 wrote to his cousin, Alfred Victor du Pont, asking for some kind of position "in a house in the West."[10]

This network between the two families served Lammot well, eventually landing him in the paper business with the du Ponts and Edgar Hounsfield, Mary Augusta's son, in Louisville. Shortly after Lammot's arrival in Louisville, Bidermann du Pont, Margaretta's son, reported in a letter to his mother that he was "much pleased" with the young man and was certain that "henceforth he can take care of himself."[11] The degree to which Lammot lived up to Bidermann du Pont's expectations is not entirely clear. In 1872, he married Ellen Newbold, daughter of Richard Smith Newbold, a Philadelphia businessman, and Ellen Da Costa, originally born in the West Indies.[12] Records show Lammot and his wife moving frequently in Louisville, perhaps for financial reasons or perhaps to accommodate the births of their three children.[13] Eventually the family left Louisville because Lammot experienced business problems, spending some time in Little Falls, Minnesota before settling in New York State in the early 1890s, where Lammot and his son went into business manufacturing boxes until they eventually moved to Wilmington in 1910. Lammot returned to the scene of his childhood, where he would live out the last seven years of his life in close proximity to his du Pont cousins and where his son would begin working for the du Pont Corporation in 1909.

In 1890, around the time her family left Louisville for Little Falls, a "Nellie La Motte" graduated from the Arlington Institute in Alexandria, Virginia, a private school for girls headed up by long-time educators, members of the Powell family, with distinction in English literature, physiology, mythology, ancient history, natural philosophy, and algebra.[14] It is probable that this is Ellen N. La Motte–she was called Nellie by members of her family and a profile of her from the 1950s states that she "attended fashionable Miss Rebecca Powell's school in Arlington, Va."[15] However, in her application to Johns Hopkins she explained that she finished her formal education at Miss Anable's Boarding and Day School in Philadelphia, an establishment that other women in the du Pont family attended and one that offered a curriculum similar to that of the Powell school. After she completed her studies, wherever she did so, she moved to the Brandywine Valley in Delaware to live with her cousin Alfred I. du Pont and his first wife until her departure for nursing school in the late 1890s.[16] This environment would serve as La Motte's social center. The earliest known photo of La Motte shows her with a group of other women dressed in costume for the Dance of Nations, in which she represented Russia, performed as part of a week-long charity event that raised money for a Delaware hospital (see Figure 2).[17] Several of the other women in the photograph are du Ponts and the rest are "society belles" who presumably served as her social network.[18]

Du Pont himself, however, was probably the most important connection she had: he came to assume the role of her father in her life despite the fact that her own father was alive at this time, and she was his favorite cousin according to one of his biographers and his third wife, Jesse Ball du Pont.[19] In the earliest surviving letter from La

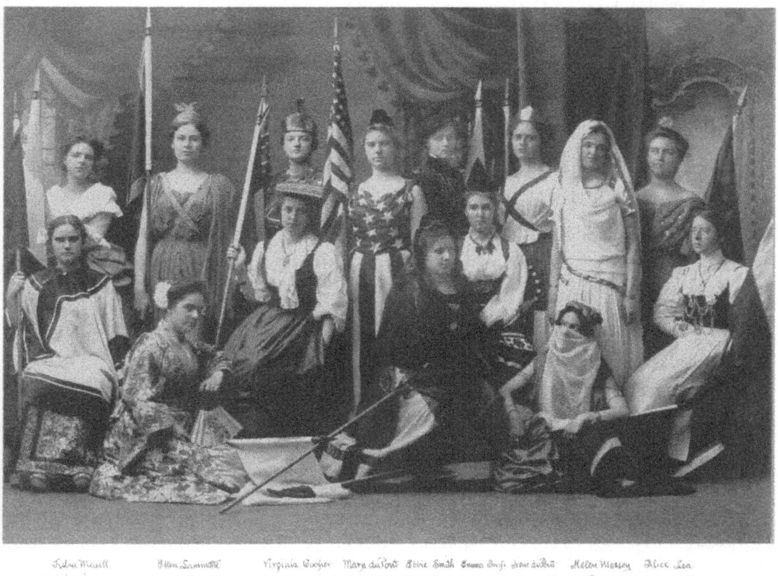

Figure 2 "Photograph of Women in Various National Costumes," 1898

Motte to du Pont, she opens with "Dearest Father"[20] and thanks him for sending her money to help defray the costs of an appendectomy she had undergone during the summer.[21] He was, according to her estimation, a "wonderful friend" and a "dear old man."[22] In this one brief letter she communicates the myriad roles he played in her life, explaining to him that her finances were in dire condition because someone had forged a check she had written, adding an extra hundred dollars to the sum, which resulted in La Motte being overdrawn at the bank. La Motte also described her efforts to help Anna Herkner, then the assistant to the chief of the Maryland Bureau of Statistics.[23] Herkner was under attack from male critics who "hate being under a woman" and La Motte was involved in trying to help her to save her position by calling on people with political sway in the region.[24] She wistfully wrote to du Pont, "[I] only wish you were in this country so that we could get you to help us out."[25] It was clearly important to La Motte to communicate to her cousin that he was a significant resource for her economically, personally, and professionally. He responded to all of her concerns, sending her a check to replace the stolen money with a word of encouragement to avoid pursuing the person who forged her check and advising her on how to handle the governor of Maryland, "a man of … high standards" in du Pont's assessment, in order to help Herkner.[26]

The rest of La Motte's correspondence with du Pont, as preserved in the Alfred I. du Pont Papers at Washington and Lee University, Lexington, VA, spans two decades and reveals that she continued to enjoy an affectionate relationship with him and often sought his advice on financial and automotive matters and delved into politics in their exchanges. In turn, he relished doling out advice on these topics as well as on other subjects on which she had not solicited his input such as healthy eating and drinking habits and why she should return to live in the United States when she made London her home in the 1920s. He also cheered on her successes and praised her work ethic, undoubtedly the reason he sent her a stipend or some kind of financial support for more than twenty years. He believed that she had "never had anything but adversity" but weathered her difficulties without complaint.[27]

Du Pont's reference could be to her constant engagement with political causes and the resistance and backlash she experienced as a result of her speeches and writing, but the comment feels more connected to her personally. Unfortunately, his letters do not elaborate on the sources of hardship in her life. An article published in *Harper's Magazine*, "The Christmas Boat," offers a tantalizing glimpse of La Motte uncharacteristically in a personal and reflective mode. The article documents her journey across the North Atlantic in mid-December on a cargo boat, having decided that there was no reason to take "a crack liner, the biggest afloat" after feeling "the spirit of adventure stirring."[28] The little boat encounters a terrible storm that lasts for days; one night she finally falls asleep in rough seas and has a dream

> in which a friend said, "Yes, I know all about it."
>
> "All about me? All about the things that hurt?"
>
> "Yes. All. Everything."
>
> "About how fearfully frightened I am? About how I try to keep up appearances and to pretend? I've been pretending so long–I'm so tired of pretending."
>
> Then in my dream I became aware of everything that had ever hurt me in my whole life–every incident, great and small, that had brought pain, humiliation, disappointment. Just everything, a whole vast piling up of all the whole pain of a lifetime, the hurt of things forgotten, put away, lived down, a vast, cumulative mass of pain, not piecemeal, but the whole of it piled together. And under the overwhelming agony of this I woke.[29]

Upon awakening, she feels "amazingly comforted" and tells herself, "That's my life … All that pain, hidden away and covered up and pushed into the background–all there, intensely acute. Unforgotten. And that is what I have been living with all these years."[30] La Motte rarely shared her intimate feelings and this scene offers an unusually raw, introspective look at the pain and frustrations that marked her life without offering any details about their origin, consequences, or her methods for coping with them.

One source of conflict and frustration is revealed in her 1898 application to the Johns Hopkins Training School for Nurses, in which she discloses that her family was opposed to her attending,[31] and it is unclear if her determining to do so had long-term effects on her relationship with them or whether the family that she says was upset included her parents with whom she had not lived since the early 1890s or her stand-in father, her cousin. Perhaps her insistence on becoming a nurse meant she had to support herself financially, and six years into her career when she was working for the Instructive Visiting Nurse Association in Baltimore, she was, according to her cousin, "hard put for money at times" and dependent on the "small sums" generated by a bond that another cousin was responsible for sending her.[32] Although she enjoyed a life full of travel and luxury when hosted by her wealthy cousins and friends, she lived modestly when on her own and worried frequently about making ends meet.[33] Her hope to become a full-time writer could not come to fruition until du Pont began giving her a stipend so she could leave her nursing position in 1913 and the modicum of financial stability it afforded her. Even then, her friendly competition with Gertrude Stein, as recorded in their correspondence, shows that earning money to support herself was a constant struggle even in her most productive and lucrative decade, the 1920s.[34] It was not until she was in her sixties that she bought her first house and lived with fewer worries about her finances. Ultimately, through her earnings, money earned on investments she made with her own funds or those given to her by her relatives, and money she inherited, she died with almost half a million dollars in assets.[35]

She was fiercely independent and may have chosen to support herself to guarantee the freedom she could never have if she were dependent on others. Although she was recognized as a "socialite" by the Philadelphia and Wilmington papers when she was in her twenties,[36] she either could not find a husband via the many social gatherings she would have been invited to or had determined she did not want a husband, the latter the more likely scenario. When she discovered she was attracted to other women and how she constructed and understood her sexuality cannot be said. Evidence that she had great passion for women only survived through the strangest turning of fate. In 2016, sixteen letters were donated to the Alan Mason Chesney Medical Archives of the Johns Hopkins Medical Institutions after they were discovered with a larger trove of letters in a goat shed in the outskirts of Berlin, Germany and donated by a descendant of the recipient, Amy Wesselhoeft von Erdberg.[37] These letters are the only time that La Motte expresses in her own words her love for a woman.

In two letters, La Motte is shockingly honest about her feelings for Louise, who is only identified by her first name. Putting such sentiments in written form no matter how trustworthy the recipient was a risk for La Motte. At the time, in 1911, she was an executive with the Baltimore Health Department, the first woman to hold such a position, and a person of note in the Baltimore community because of her lecturing on the subject of tuberculosis and her participation in the suffrage movement–both of which had resulted in her being mentioned on many occasions in the local papers. She was putting her professional life in peril and her relationships with her family at stake by expressing her intense passion for Louise in a way that could easily have been shared with others. Clearly, she trusted Wesselhoeft von Erdberg completely and was at a point in her life when she was willing to take enormous chances for the person she loved. Unfortunately, Louise was not ready to risk bringing shame to her family and being cut off by them: she rejected La Motte's entreaties to leave with her for Europe, where they could start life anew.[38]

Two years later, La Motte left for Europe, where she set out to make a life for herself without Louise. By January 1915, she was on very familiar terms with Emily Rockwell Crane Chadbourne, whom she called E. C., an abbreviation that in the context of her diary from that year is a sign of familiarity.[39] There is no indication of how the two women met, but it was very likely at Stein's.[40] Chadbourne was the daughter of the wealthy Chicago-based industrialist Richard Teller Crane, who made a fortune manufacturing plumbing supplies. She married Thomas L. Chadbourne, a lawyer, in 1896 and they divorced nine years later after she charged him with desertion.[41] When she filed for divorce, she was already living abroad in Europe, where she still was in 1913 when La Motte moved to London, then Paris. Chadbourne was an art collector who purchased modern works by Matisse and Cézanne, amongst others, that she later donated to various museums, most generously to the Chicago Art Institute in the 1920s. She was also an avid collector of decorative arts that made their way to these same museums.[42]

Chadbourne's niece, Margaret C.-L. Gildea, a psychiatrist, in 1978, fifteen years after the death of her aunt, sent the Chicago Historical Society an account of Chadbourne's life to accompany the donation of a trove of papers related to Chadbourne and the Crane Company. In it, she describes Chadbourne as being "unprepared for matrimony" and "no good at wifely duties."[43] The couple never had children, although Thomas Chadbourne would later have a son with his second wife, all of which implies that she may have resisted intimacy with her husband. After the divorce, she never remarried and maintained a relationship with La Motte from probably 1913 or 1914 until La Motte's death in 1961. What they meant to each other is difficult to assess since they left no letters between them to reveal the content and nature of their correspondence when they were separated, which they often were as they lived in different homes, usually located in close proximity, and went on trips without each other. In her correspondence with her cousin, La Motte maintained a formality about "Mrs. Chadbourne," as she and du Pont frequently referred to her, that is absent in her communication with Stein and Toklas. For example, in one letter to Toklas, La Motte tells her that "Em was awfully sick … and I was terribly worried" and "nearly distracted" by fear she might not recover, expressing a sense of urgency about her health that would have been surprising in letters to her cousin.[44]

Stein and Toklas, as Macleod writes, "were magnets for American women who went abroad to reformulate themselves in the first decades of the twentieth century."[45] Like many others, La Motte admired Stein's intellectual and artistic abilities and saw her as a person who, like her du Pont cousin, was a good source of advice when she had a big decision to make, for example, about whether to go to Serbia in 1915.[46] In the 1910s, in the few letters and postcards that survive, La Motte refers to her as "Miss Stein" but in the 1920s she had switched to "Dear Gertrude," a more familiar mode of address that Chadbourne adopted around the same time as well, reflecting an evolution in the nature of the women's friendship. Macleod comments that Stein and Toklas were also models in particular for women who "wanted to liberate their sexuality. Especially after 1914, when [Stein] began to live openly in a lesbian relationship with Alice B. Toklas."[47] La Motte undoubtedly would have found Stein's ability to have the kind of relationship she had ardently wished for with Louise something to admire. She did not, however, engage in a similarly open relationship with Chadbourne, who was raised in a religious family and was presumably unwilling to expose her relationship with La Motte in a direct way, something they must have come to terms with together given they enjoyed the next fifty years in a consistent and from all available signs mutually beneficial relationship.

Whereas La Motte, as expressed in the letters to Wesselhoeft von Erdberg, forthrightly identified her passionate love for Louise and understood the risks associated with declaring that love, it is unclear if she experienced the same intense desire for Chadbourne. It is also unknown how Chadbourne conceptualized her feelings for La Motte, though it is evident that she leaned on her to take care of things like packing up her apartments and scouting places for her to live and later in life giving her financial advice. Whether they defined their relationship as lesbian is something that will probably never be determined. Smith-Rosenberg has analyzed how "nineteenth-century American society did not taboo close female relationships but rather recognized them as a socially viable form of human contact–and, as such, acceptable throughout a woman's life."[48] Born in the early 1870s, Chadbourne and La Motte would have been socialized in environments in which close female relationships were important parts of the middle- and upper-class lives they led, and which had more latitude in terms of physical and emotional closeness.[49] It was, for example, typical for girls to share a bed and exchange embraces without censure.[50] La Motte used terms of endearment, such as "my precious Amy", in her letters to Wesselhoeft von Erdberg and talked about a "honeymoon" they were supposed to take, using language that crosses over into territory that would now be viewed as romantic. In an essay reflecting on the process of writing a biography of Molly Dewson and contextualizing her relationship with her companion of many years, Polly Porter, Susan Ware deliberates "to what extent the label 'lesbianism' is appropriate for understanding the Porter–Dewson relationship," a question that applies equally to that of La Motte and Chadbourne.[51] They left no letters testifying to their feelings for each other, and without that evidence it is impossible to say whether they shared intimacy beyond the emotional. Ware's conclusion that knowledge of whether Porter and Dewson were physically intimate is not "necessarily central to our understanding of their relationship" is also applicable to La Motte and Chadbourne.[52] The two were bonded in essential ways and functioned much like a married couple, albeit one that took up separate residences.

La Motte certainly depended on close female friendships and is part of the group of women Ware says "built their emotional lives around other women rather than men."[53] She explains, in a statement that fully applies to La Motte, that "the participation of many women in public life in the early twentieth century was characterized by a similar congruence between informal friendships and public activism. The key instruments were networks that brought together reformers, political activists, and traditional women's organizations on issues of common concern. These networks maximized women's influence and offered a powerful tool with which to influence public policy."[54] La Motte had close relationships with women that encompassed the personal and professional, including with nurse Carolyn Conant van Blarcom, a 1901 Johns Hopkins graduate. They were supervising nurses at Johns Hopkins at the same time and then two years later worked together in St. Louis for a year. Presumably, they had a good friendship in order for La Motte to take up residence and a position in a new city. La Motte returned to Baltimore to work with Mary E. Lent, an 1895 graduate of Johns Hopkins and the head of the Instructive Visiting Nurse Association of Baltimore. The two were collaborators, co-presenting and publishing on the best methods, seen as controversial by other practitioners, of combating tuberculosis. They shared a strong commitment to advocating for the vote for women and traveled to Europe together. Their relationship probably transcended friendship, as La Motte suggests in a letter to Wesselhoeft von Erdberg when she refers to her relationship with "Mary."[55] For La Motte, the boundaries between personal and professional and romantic love and friendship may have been porous.

However La Motte and these women intersected, their relationships were important to her intellectual growth, allowing her to test, further, and prove her ideas and interests alongside and sometimes in conflict with the women. Nursing, at the time an all-female world, helped her to form relationships that bridged nursing and suffrage. Many of the women of Johns Hopkins were active in the suffrage campaign and were well prepared to take on speaking in public and writing editorials in favor of the vote. Their nursing careers had readied them to find their voices and confidence, whether it be when speaking on behalf of nursing or suffrage, and they relied on their nursing networks to promote the suffrage cause, stumping at some of the same meetings and combining their efforts to write for publications like the *New Voter*, of which Mary Bartlett Dixon, a 1903 Johns Hopkins Training School for Nurses graduate and friend of La Motte, was the Associate

Editor, with La Motte a contributor representing the Just Government League of Maryland. Later, La Motte served as a contributing editor, as did Dr. Florence B. Sabin, a graduate of the Johns Hopkins medical school, for *Maryland Suffrage News*, of which Edith Houghton Hooker, who attended medical school at Johns Hopkins, served as Editor-in-Chief.

These professional women associated with Johns Hopkins were energized by the national and international suffrage movements gaining momentum across the globe. In the United States, by 1910 women had gained the right to vote in a handful of western territories and states,[56] inspiring women in the other parts of the country to launch their own efforts. Progress was slow, however, in part because of differing views regarding the best method by which women could win the vote: through a constitutional amendment, the path forward favored by the National Woman Suffrage Association, formed in 1869, or by a state-by-state approach backed by the American Woman Suffrage Association, also formed in 1869.[57] Even with the merging of the two groups into the National American Woman Suffrage Association (NAWSA) in 1890, tensions in the organization remained high because of disagreement over which method was the best way forward, although NAWSA would eventually, under the leadership of President Carrie Chapman Catt, focus on the importance of winning state-level suffrage before striving for a federal amendment, and from the early 1890s to 1913 the attempt to win a federal amendment languished as intense campaigning at the state level was taking place across the country,[58] including Maryland, where, from 1909 to 1913, La Motte was increasingly engaged in the suffrage fight, at first focusing on winning municipal suffrage, a position she eventually disowned.[59]

La Motte's interest in suffrage would evolve to include an interest in militant tactics, buoyed no doubt by reading about the upsurge in such activity via sympathetic publications like the *Woman's Journal* after Emmeline Pankhurst formed the Women's Social and Political Union (WSPU) in 1903.[60] American activists such as Harriet Stanton Blatch, who returned to the United States in 1902 after advocating for the vote for women during the two decades she lived in England, brought new energy to the fight and had relationships with militant advocates like Pankhurst, sponsoring her speaking tour in the United

States in 1909.[61] These visits gave women like La Motte "an opportunity to honor the suffragettes, to hear about their methods firsthand, and to win more attention and support for their own efforts."[62] These methods incited La Motte's curiosity, but she also attended lectures by English suffragists who eschewed militant actions, such as Ethel Snowden.[63] Ultimately, however, she chose to investigate militancy when she took a leave from her nursing position in June 1913 to travel to England to investigate their methods.

The militant movement under the auspices of Emmeline Pankhurst and the WSPU had been increasing its use of violent and disruptive tactics over 1913, including the launching of an arson campaign in January that continued throughout that winter and spring.[64] On June 4, 1913, suffragette Emily Wilding Davison threw herself in front of King George V's horse at the Derby in Epsom and died several days later on June 8 from injuries incurred as a result of her actions.[65] She was treated as a martyr at her death and thousands of suffragettes walked through the streets of London to St. George's Church before her body was sent back to Northumberland for burial.[66] Although her actions, which were not sanctioned by the WSPU, did not have a long-term political impact on progress toward acquiring the vote, they did show that "at least one of their women would give her life for the Cause and raised the possibility there were more waiting in the wings" and brought increased attention and criticism to the movement.[67] La Motte arrived in England at the end of June in time for July and August, downtimes for WSPU activities,[68] but attended London meetings to gather information to report back in a series of articles for the *Sun*.[69]

This accumulated experience prepared La Motte to engage fully with the anti-opium crusade after she witnessed the devastating effects of the drug while traveling in Asia from the summer of 1916 to that of 1917. Already well versed in the means and methods of campaigning, she immediately set to work publishing articles, books, fiction and non-fiction, and eventually giving talks intended to mobilize readers and listeners to demand that the countries, particularly Great Britain, benefiting from the lax regulation of the opium trade, reform their policies. Combating the enormous profits reaped by European countries in the exploitation of colonized people through the laws regulating opium was an almost hopeless cause. Although La Motte's reputation today rests in large part on her writing about World War One, she devoted two decades to the anti-opium crusade and won international recognition in the form of the Order for Merit from the Japanese Red Cross in 1918 and the Lin Tse Hsu Memorial Medal from China in 1930. She wrote more on this topic than any other, and engagement with this subject led her to expand her networks to encompass politicians and activists in the United States, Europe, and Asia as she tried to build alliances to promote the cause.

The Great Depression curtailed La Motte's political activism in the early 1930s, resulting in her returning to the United States to live permanently. She settled in Washington, DC, where she thrived on the political scene, investing in real estate in the Georgetown area of the city and enjoying her extensive network of friends. Although her days of hard campaigning were over and she published her last article in 1934, she maintained intellectual interests that she fostered by keeping herself engaged with her community and her friends. In a letter written in 1957, just four years before the end of her life, La Motte recounted a meeting with a friend in which they "talked as we have never talked before–about death and dying," leading her to observe, "It is sad to see the old lions go down."[70] An "old lion" herself, La Motte was nearing her own death. What she thought about at the end of her long and productive life can only be imagined. She surely looked upon her decades of writing, speeches, and activism on topics as varied as tuberculosis, suffrage, and opium with a sense of pride. Born at a time when women were not expected or encouraged to participate in public debate about medical and political matters, she found her voice and made an imprint in these fields, leaving behind an impressive record as a nurse, writer, and activist.

Notes

1 The Alan Mason Chesney Medical Archives of the Johns Hopkins Medical Institutions, Baltimore, MD (hereafter JHMI), "Ellen N. La Motte, Alumni Questionnaire," Biographical Files, 1951.

2 *Ibid.*

3 "Pioneers in Public Health: Ellen N. La Motte," *Trained Nurse and Hospital Review* 81:3 (September 1928).

4 *Ibid.*

5 JHMI, "Alumni Questionnaire."

6 The family began using a different spelling for their last name, changing it from Lammot to the original French La Motte, at some point, probably in the late nineteenth century. See E. C. Silver, *Sketches of the New Church in America on a Background of Civic and Social Life* (Boston, MA: New Church Union, 1920), p. 311.

7 Historical Society of Pennsylvania, Philadelphia, PA, Historic Pennsylvania Church and Town Records, Reel 776.

8 Delaware Public Archives, Dover, DE, Wilmington, Delaware Death Registers, 1849, RG 1500.061.

9 Anthony F.C. Wallace, *Rockdale: The Growth of an American Village in the Early Industrial Revolution* (1978; repr., Lincoln, NE: University of Nebraska Press, 2005), p. 94.

10 Margaretta E. du Pont Coleman Papers (hereafter MDPC), Box 13, Hagley Museum and Library, Wilmington, DE, "Ferdinand Lammot to Alfred V. du Pont," August 11, 1865. Some of the history of the du Pont family in Louisville is fleshed out in T. J. Mullin, "The du Ponts in Kentucky: Louisville's Central Park, the Southern Exposition, and an Entrepreneurial Spirit," TopSCHOLAR, DLSC Faculty Publications Paper 18, last modified 2009, accessed 19 September 2012, http://digitalcommons.wku.edu/dlsc_fac_pub/18.

11 MDPC, Box 7, "Bidermann du Pont to Margaretta E. Lammot du Pont," December 17, 1865.

12 Richard S. Newbold's sister was Mary B. Newbold. She married John Singer and was grandmother to the painter John Singer Sargent (1856–1925), making La Motte his distant cousin. She was aware of the relation as attested to in a letter she wrote to a friend referring to "her revered and famous cousin"; see JHMI, Ellen N. La Motte Collection, "La Motte to Amy Wesselhoeft von Erdberg," May 6, 1914. She also mentioned that his painting had been "hacked," a reference to an attack by Mary Wood, an English suffragette, on the painting at the Royal Academy Exhibition on May 4, 1914. See Thomas J. Otten, "Slashing Henry James," *Yale Journal of Criticism* 13:2 (2000), pp. 293–320, for a brief account of the attack.

13 Between 1873, the year of Ellen La Motte's birth, and 1891, when *Caron's Annual Directory of the City of Louisville* lists Ferdinand Lammot as having moved to Little Falls, Minnesota, Lammot lived at eight different addresses. The family grew when La Motte's sister, Augusta, was born in 1876–she died in 1954–and her brother, Ferdinand, was born in 1879; he died in 1961.

14 "Commencement Exercises," *Alexandria Gazette and Virginia Advertiser* (June 24, 1890), p. 2.

15 Jane Eads, "The Washington Scene," *Town Talk* (December 6, 1951), p. 8.

16 Marquis James, *Alfred I. duPont: The Family Rebel* (Indianapolis, IN: Bobbs-Merrill, 1941), p. 96.

17 Newspaper coverage of the event also indicates that she took part in a Georgia cakewalk orchestrated by her cousin, Alfred I. du Pont. See "Buds, Belles and Gallants Make a Success of the Temple of Fame," *Philadelphia Inquirer* (October 30, 1898), p. 29. The photograph is in the Hagley Library and Museum.
18 *Ibid.*
19 Joseph Frazier Wall, *Alfred I. du Pont: The Man and His Family* (New York: Oxford University Press, 1990), p. 434. Jesse Ball du Pont Papers (hereafter JBDP), Washington and Lee University, Lexington, VA, "Jesse Ball du Pont to Ellen N. La Motte," December 19, 1929.
20 Alfred I. du Pont Papers (hereafter AID), Washington and Lee University, Lexington, VA, "Ellen N. La Motte to Alfred I. du Pont," October 4, 1912.
21 "Miss La Motte under Knife," *Sun* (July 21, 1912), p. 12. This and all subsequent references to the *Sun* are to the *Baltimore Sun*.
22 AID, "La Motte to du Pont," October 4, 1912.
23 "Pioneer Maryland Social Worker Dies," *Evening Sun* (December 4, 1959), p. 10. This and all subsequent references to the *Evening Sun* are to the *Baltimore Evening Sun*.
24 AID, "La Motte to du Pont," October 4, 1912.
25 *Ibid.*
26 *Ibid.*
27 AID, "Alfred I. du Pont to Ellen N. La Motte," April 29, 1932.
28 Ellen N. La Motte, "The Christmas Boat," *Harper's Magazine* (March 1930), p. 490.
29 *Ibid.*, pp. 495–496.
30 *Ibid.*, p. 496.
31 See Chapter 1 for a discussion of her application to Johns Hopkins.
32 AID, "Alfred I du Pont to T.C. du Pont," March 25, 1908.
33 These kinds of concerns prompted her to take the cargo boat featured in "The Christmas Boat."
34 Gertrude Stein and Alice B. Toklas Papers (hereafter GSABTP), Yale Collection of American Literature, Beinecke Rare Book and Manuscript Library, Yale University, New Haven, CT, "La Motte to Stein, 13 February 1929."
35 Probate Court, District of Columbia, "Inventory of the Goods, Chattels, and Personal Estate of Ellen Newbold La Motte."
36 "Tete-a-Tete," *Times* (Philadelphia) (April 12, 1898), p. 6.
37 Caroline H. Williams describes the origin of the letters and her family's papers in *Lives in Letters: A New England Family, 1870–2000* (Createspace, 2015).
38 See Chapter 2 for more detailed discussion of the letters.
39 Private Collection, Ellen N. La Motte, Unpublished Diary (hereafter Diary), "January 13, 1915."

40 Macleod says that "Chadbourne's introduction to Stein had been brokered by La Motte," but she does not provide a source to support this assertion; see D. Macleod, *Enchanted Lives, Enchanted Objects: American Women Collectors and the Making of Culture, 1800–1940* (Berkeley, CA: University of California Press, 2008), p. 194.
41 "Sues to Quit Chadbourne," *Chicago Tribune* (June 28, 1905), p. 9.
42 See Macleod, *Enchanted Lives*, and R. S. Nelson, "The Art Collecting of Emily Crane Chadbourne and the Absence of Byzantine Art in Chicago," in C. Nielsen (ed.), *To Inspire and Instruct: A History of Medieval Art in Midwestern Museums* (Newcastle upon Tyne: Cambridge Scholars Publishing, 2008), pp. 131–148, for more on Chadbourne's art collecting.
43 Chicago History Museum (hereafter CHM), Crane Family and Lillie Family Papers, 1833–1978 (bulk 1890s–1960s), "Essay by Margaret Crane Lillie Gildea Discussing Crane Family Relations with the Crane Company, with Emphasis on Emily Crane Chadbourne (1871–1964), written 1978."
44 GSABTP, "La Motte to Toklas," April 10, 1926.
45 Macleod, *Enchanted Lives*, p. 176.
46 See La Motte, Diary, "January 18, 1915." This conversation is undoubtedly the origin of Stein's comment that La Motte was "gun shy"; see Gertrude Stein, *The Autobiography of Alice B. Toklas* (New York: Vintage, 1990), p. 158. For more on the subject, see Chapter 3. In a letter, La Motte apologizes for not being able to see her and says she wants to get her opinion on several matters; see "La Motte to Stein 25 November 1914," GSABTP.
47 Macleod, *Enchanted Lives*, p. 176.
48 Carroll Smith-Rosenberg, "The Female World of Love and Ritual: Relations between Women in Nineteenth-Century America," in J. W. Leavitt (ed.), *Women and Health in America* (Madison, WI: Wisconsin University Press, 1984), p. 81.
49 Of interest is one of the friendships Smith-Rosenberg analyzes in her chapter, that between Clementina Smith (1814–1888) and Sophie M. Du Pont (1810–1888), relatives of La Motte. They are women who would have fostered the kind of close female bonds in their younger relatives that they experienced and valued. See Smith-Rosenberg, "The Female World," pp. 70–89.
50 *Ibid.*, p. 79.
51 Susan Ware, "Unlocking the Porter–Dewson Partnership: A Challenge for the Feminist Biographer," in S. Alpern, Joyce Antler, Elisabeth I. Perry, and Ingrid W. Scobie (eds), *The Challenge of Feminist Biography: Writing the Lives of Modern American Women* (Chicago: University of Illinois Press, 1992), p. 58.
52 *Ibid.*, p. 59.
53 *Ibid.*, p. 53.
54 *Ibid.*

55 JHMI, Ellen N. La Motte Collection, "La Motte to Amy Wesselhoeft von Erdberg," May 6, 1914. See Chapters 1 and 2 for discussion of La Motte and Lent's collaboration in the anti-tuberculosis and suffrage campaigns.
56 See Eleanor Flexner, *Century of Struggle: The Woman's Rights Movement in the United States* (New York: Atheneum, 1970), pp. 156–163, and Rebecca Edwards, "Pioneers at the Polls: Woman Suffrage in the West," in J. Baker (ed.), *Votes for Women: The Struggle for Suffrage Revisited* (Oxford: Oxford University Press, 2002), pp. 90–101, for a discussion of the vote for women in the western states.
57 See Flexner, *Century of Struggle*, for an assessment of the differing views of the two organizations.
58 Corrine M. McConnaughy in *The Woman Suffrage Movement in America: A Reassessment* (Cambridge: Cambridge University Press, 2013) analyzes the importance of legislative work done at the state level that resulted in enfranchising women.
59 See Chapter 2 for a discussion of La Motte's suffrage activities and shifting views.
60 Bolt explains that Lucy Stone shared new militant techniques as early as 1906 in the *Woman's Journal*; see Christine Bolt, "America and the Pankhursts," in Baker (ed.), *Votes for Women*, p. 152.
61 Ellen Carol DuBois, "The Next Generation: Harriet Stanton Blatch and Grassroots Politics," in Baker (ed.), *Votes for Women*, p. 161.
62 Bolt, "America and the Pankhursts," p. 152.
63 "Mrs. Snowden Eloquent," *Sun* (November 28, 1909), p. 12.
64 Andrew Rosen, *Rise Up, Women! The Militant Campaign of the Women's Social and Political Union 1903–1914* (London: Routledge and Kegan Paul, 1974), p. 189.
65 For a succinct biography of Davison, see Elizabeth Crawford, *The Women's Suffrage Movement: A Reference Guide 1866–1928* (London: UCL Press, 1999), pp. 159–163.
66 *Ibid.*, pp. 200–201.
67 Diane Atkinson, *Rise Up, Women! The Remarkable Lives of the Suffragettes* (London: Bloomsbury, 2018), 417.
68 Rosen, *Rise Up, Women!*, p. 202.
69 See Chapter 2 for analysis of La Motte's suffrage work and writings.
70 Howry Family Collection, Archives and Special Collections, J. D. Williams Library, University of Mississippi, Oxford, MS, "Ellen N. La Motte to Mary Howry," September 26, 1957.

1

Becoming professionalized: La Motte and nursing, 1898–1913

The path La Motte traveled during the course of her life becomes visible just after she took her first step toward independence from her family and began developing a professional life for herself. That moment came in 1898 when she applied to the Johns Hopkins Training School for Nurses. Georgina Caird Ross, the second assistant in the training school at the time of La Motte's application, observes in notes left in her student record, that La Motte was "most attractive, very handsome & ladylike."[1] Johns Hopkins was distinct from many training schools in the late nineteenth century in that it attracted women who tended to be well educated and from families with some social status.[2] La Motte was undoubtedly very much the kind of woman the training school was eager to admit: she was white, middle class, and had important family connections.

Like many women applying to Johns Hopkins,[3] La Motte experienced conflict with her family over her decision. After being accepted she had to defer her entrance, explaining in a letter that "my family objects bitterly to my going to the hospital, and have demanded of me that I wait six months before going."[4] In her entreaty to be allowed the deferral, La Motte clarified that if she did not wait, she was in danger of having "an utter and absolute break in all my relations with my people–a complete burning of ships."[5] Whatever pressure her family brought to bear during this period of time, by November 1898, a mere two months later, the *Morning News* of Wilmington, Delaware shared her impending departure in a rather overwrought announcement:

> 'Twas ever woman's province to lend her tender care to the ills and weaknesses of mankind. No lovelier woman is ever drawn than that of the sweet-faced nurse, administering comfort to the suffering. Since Florence

> Nightingale gave her life and tender regard to suffering humanity, the name of nurse has had a halo of romance about it. Many society girls feeling that the hollow round of balls, dinners and receptions, and the mad vortex of Frivol Palace did not satisfy them, has given her life to others, and taken upon herself the arduous duties of nursedom. One of our belles and favorites in Vanity Fair has said good-bye to tulle and dancing slippers this winter and adopted the apron and cap of the hospital nurse. Miss Ellen La Motte left last week for a hospital, where she will take a three years' course in the science of nursing. It is likely she will take her first instructions at Johns Hopkins Hospital, Baltimore.[6]

Whether or not this highly romanticized version of nursing matched La Motte's expectations of what awaited her, she "left a P.P.C. card" with the local gossip columnists in late November,[7] signaling her intentions to be absent from the balls, luncheons, and teas she had frequented for some years to begin the training course soon thereafter, determined, as Ross recorded in her notes taken during their initial interview, to "make something out of her life."[8]

In her formal written letter of application, La Motte stated that she "never had any occupation at all,"[9] a situation she was willing to take dramatic action to correct, even at the risk of inciting serious disagreements with her family. The prospect of familial discord was worth it, for La Motte chose well when she decided upon the training school at Johns Hopkins. By the late nineteenth century, the professionalization of nursing was well under way, and it offered her the opportunity to learn patient care while being exposed to the legacy of influential women who were elevating the status of nursing and carving out careers as activists and reformers.

An examination of La Motte's movements and early writings (1901–1906) reveals that she was keen to establish her professional footing by sharing her scholarly interests through publication and developing her career in dynamic ways. What is less easily accessible is her personal development through these years, when she undoubtedly flourished as a result of being surrounded by other intelligent, curious women who wanted to establish themselves in respectable nursing careers. There is no surviving personal evidence in the form of letters or diaries to indicate how she initially responded to the excitement and energy of this stimulating environment. As a few sources show, she thrived enough in nursing school to win a scholarship for her intermediate year, a sign that by then she was

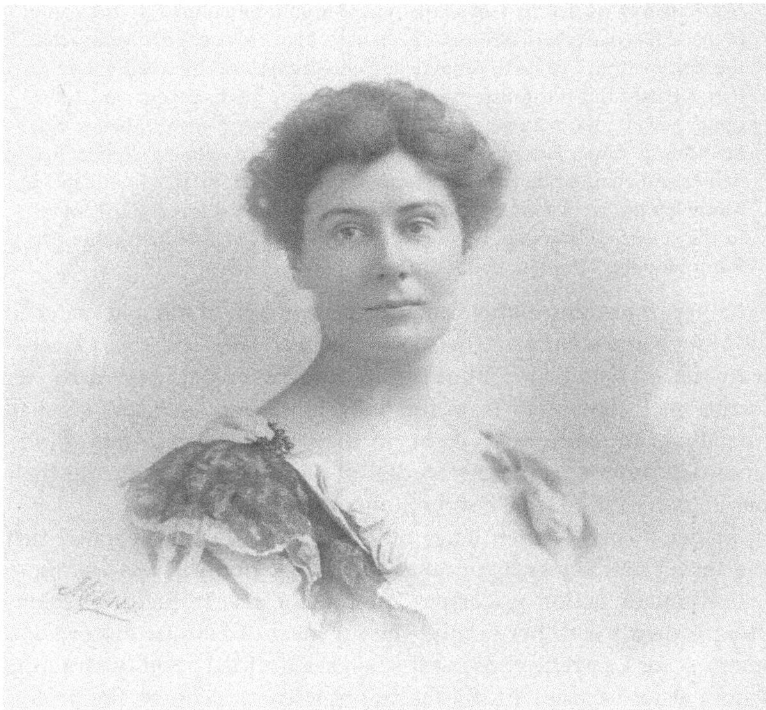

Figure 3 Portrait of La Motte, *c.* 1902

distinguishing herself amongst her peers.[10] Then, after her graduation in May 1902, free of obligations, she moved and changed jobs several times: initially working as a supervising nurse for the year 1902–1903 at the Johns Hopkins Hospital and Training School,[11] she then left for Italy, where she took a break before assuming charge of a private patient,[12] presumably through her connections with another Johns Hopkins nursing student. La Motte's address during her stay in Florence was that of C. H. Fitzgerald,[13] the father of Alice Fitzgerald, a Johns Hopkins graduate who began her studies in 1902 though she had to interrupt them to return to Italy–perhaps providing La Motte the opportunity to set herself up in private duty nursing in Europe.[14]

By early spring of 1904, La Motte was back in the United States and soon departed for St. Louis, where she took a position at St. Luke's Hospital as an operating nurse.[15] She went to St. Luke's either at or around the same time as a fellow Johns Hopkins graduate, Carolyn Van Blarcom, who graduated from the training school in 1901 and was appointed superintendent of nurses at the hospital, described as "under the auspices of the Episcopal Church though undenominational in its work" and housed in "new quarters ... with about one hundred and ten beds" and "equipped in the most modern manner as regards heating, ventilation, and plumbing, with excellent electric lighting and its own ice-plant."[16] La Motte and Van Blarcom resigned from St. Luke's at the same time, with Van Blarcom taking a rest due to poor health and La Motte commencing, in June 1905, the work that would occupy her for the next eight years.[17] Developing her public voice throughout this period, La Motte produced multiple articles exploring the history of various European hospitals and nursing practices abroad. These fledgling efforts furnish a glimpse of the intellectual and professional interests that absorbed La Motte and shaped her future scholarly concerns as she began wage-earning for the first time in her late twenties.

La Motte began publishing as early as 1901, when "Early Struggles with Contagion" appeared in the *American Journal of Nursing*. The article documents La Motte's interest in medical history, particularly the origins of diseases. To open, she describes how virulent diseases such as leprosy and the plague "were combated only by the religious rites and impotent methods of ignorance."[18] Published four years before she would embark on a career in tuberculosis nursing, the statement points to an issue which La Motte would spend much of her professional life as a nurse advocating: fighting ignorance and disease through education. Her faith in science combined with the forces of education led her to declare at the end of the article that "the natural growth of better sanitation and hygiene [are] bringing us within sight of the day when those diseases which for centuries have held humanity in subjection shall themselves be brought into subjection and under control."[19]

This optimistic view of humanity's power to subdue and manage threatening diseases would eventually be tested and tempered by her experiences with the urban poor in Baltimore, yet her last written statement on tuberculosis, her book *The Tuberculosis Nurse*, echoed this position fourteen years later; in it she theorizes that "the sole way of overcoming it [tuberculosis] is to overcome the ignorance concerning its nature, its transmissibility, and the means by which it is spread."[20] Although the methods she promoted to eradicate ignorance would undergo permutations during her career, La Motte steadfastly perceived her goal as a nurse to be combating and curing ignorance.

Before La Motte became intensely focused on the tuberculosis problem between 1905 and 1912, she sought opportunities to share her research interests. Her articles published between 1904 and 1906 are concerned with describing hospitals and nursing practices in France and Italy. Her attention in these pieces tends to be on evaluating hospitals and nursing staffs according to the standards she learned at Johns Hopkins, revealing the degree to which she had internalized the professionalism espoused there. These concerns demonstrate that she was well schooled in the debates about the professionalization of nursing and that she viewed her writings as an opportunity to make the case for the value of a trained nurse. Her overview of the Galliera Hospital in "A Modern Italian Hospital" reveals some of her professional preoccupations. At one point, while describing the layout of the hospital, about which she is generally positive, she incredulously explains that in the head sister's office there is a window from which the sister could see all that happened in the main ward. She remarks, "One could imagine the glances that might be fired through this little port-hole–also having to work with such a veiled, omniscient eye fixed constantly upon one!"[21] Clearly, the idea of being under invisible surveillance is something against which La Motte chafed and offers an indication of her thirst for independence, something she would seek by going into public health nursing, recognized as the type of nursing that allowed the most autonomy.[22]

La Motte's subsequent remarks, however, clarify why such a window might be necessary when she explains that the "actual nursing care" was left to "men and women of the lower classes."[23] These "Infirmarists" receive some minimal training by doctors, "a beginning step in the right direction" and "a recognition on the physician's part of a requirement for nursing skill and efficiency that has hitherto never been felt."[24] However, it is questionable whether potential patients would value any effort to train such amateurs.

"Private Nursing in Italy" describes a female patient who used nurses as servants, ignorant of the medical knowledge they could employ to assist her. La Motte analyzes the patient's behavior by explaining, "A nurse of my caliber she could not understand and had no use for–she preferred to order a servant and to ask of a medical man."[25] La Motte sees this woman as an example of "a type–a type of the public here which is yet uneducated as to what offices and intelligences may be combined in the person of a *trained* nurse."[26] The effort to introduce trained nursing into this environment would necessarily fail unless the patient too could be trained to understand and use the abilities of experts such as La Motte, discarding the perception of the nurse as a "domestic servant."[27]

La Motte further distances the nurse from this image of a domestic drudge when she praises the "directress" of the Hôpital Général in Rheims, France, whom she describes as "a woman of great executive ability."[28] She applauds the woman for organizing "as a first step in the reform [of the hospital] a violent crusade against dirt."[29] Having visited the hospital two years earlier, La Motte gives it high marks for having made enormous progress, in large part due to the organizational skills of the aforementioned woman. Her attention to this aspect of hospital management is telling; La Motte, intelligent and ambitious, had plans for her own career that would combine the practical training she received as a student at Johns Hopkins and the executive ability that she saw in the leading women in nursing, many of whom were at one time associated with Johns Hopkins, such as Isabel Hampton Robb, Lavinia Dock, and Adelaide Nutting, whose writings and advocacy in the realm of public health undoubtedly affected the trajectory of La Motte's career.[30]

Another primary concern in these early articles is to offer advice to those wishing to work in Europe, reporting on the practicalities that nurses would need to think about before embarking on such an endeavor. La Motte emerges as a credible professional who has the authority bestowed on her by her Johns Hopkins credentials as well as those of a hands-on practitioner. She explains her decision to nurse in Italy, commenting that "there are those of us … who get tired of working in our own particular town, and who think that nursing in a foreign country, in a different atmosphere, and amid novel surroundings would be equally profitable and perhaps more diverting."[31] This passage communicates the restlessness that marked La Motte's life, a quality that pushed her to leave Baltimore, where undoubtedly she could have found work with her education and connections. It also suggests that having graduated at most only two years earlier, she already had tired of the professional opportunities afforded by that community, preferring to strike out on her own to fashion a life that would expose her to the unfamiliar. In the event other women were seeking similar opportunities, La Motte methodically takes the reader through the challenges of finding patients, ideally American tourists who are willing to pay "twenty-one to twenty-five dollars a week."[32] She enumerates other challenges, both financial and linguistic, to the American nurse, stripping the prospects of nursing abroad of any unmitigated glamor and presenting the realities of finding patients, paying for necessities, and negotiating language barriers. All these obstacles were worth overcoming, according to her final enthusiastic remarks, in which she explains, "The hours off duty or between cases I shall make no effort to describe. They are the hours that make everything worth while–they are the hours for which one comes abroad!"[33] Although La Motte took great pleasure in employing her professional skills in this foreign locale, she did leave Italy, perhaps because of the financial realities she outlined, and returned to the United States, where, a year later, she embarked on the next stage of her career, ultimately creating a name for herself as an expert in the tuberculosis crusade.

La Motte's first step was accepting a position with the Baltimore Instructive Visiting Nurse Association (hereafter IVNA) in 1905. Grace Osler, the wife of Dr. William Osler, a physician at Johns Hopkins Hospital and a member of the faculty of the school of medicine from 1888 to 1905, was inspired by the Tuberculosis Exposition held in Baltimore in 1904 to raise funds to support a nurse dedicated to tuberculosis nursing for the IVNA.[34] La Motte took the position more than a year after the first nurse specializing in tuberculosis care had started taking charge of such patients. She immediately began writing about the work being done in this area, publishing articles in medical journals as well as those devoted to philanthropy and reform. In so doing, she entered into conversations with other nurses who were similarly engaged in efforts to combat disease and to carry out sweeping social reforms.[35] These articles trace the arc followed by her positions regarding the prevention of tuberculosis. She initially promoted the promise of education as the most important tool in the campaign against the disease, then rejected the belief that most patients could be educated, thus necessitating the intervention of the state and implementation of a system of surveillance that would oversee and put under its control the tubercular bodies of Baltimore.

In a 1905 article, the first devoted to her new area of concern, La Motte explains that for those stricken with the disease "very little real nursing care … may be given."[36] She qualifies her statement by explaining that "consumption is a chronic rather than an acute disease, and until the last very few patients are confined to bed," in which case the little nursing that could be done for them, such as "a bed bath [and] alcohol rub," could be provided by a family member.[37] At first glance, La Motte appears to be undermining the highly trained professional nurse's importance by arguing that the kind of care required by tuberculosis patients could be administered by the untrained. However, she describes a more elevated task the nurse has to carry out: "The greater part of the work … is instructive and preventive, and means carrying the campaign of education and enlightenment directly into those households in which the disease originates and from which it is disseminated."[38] In this comment, La Motte aligns herself with the vision of the visiting nurse as a "missionary of health" who would "translate the knowledge of scientific medicine into concepts of disease prevention and personal responsibility for health."[39]

The targets of her educational campaign are those living "in unsanitary, overcrowded, and poverty-stricken households," including "domestic servants, laundresses, [and] dressmakers."[40] Her language reveals the crusading spirit that characterized the approach to eradicating tuberculosis taken by many health-care professionals. She explains that "the visits of the nurse to these households means [*sic*] bringing the knowledge of sanitary living and preventive care directly into the homes of the people most in need of such knowledge."[41] La Motte expresses faith in the power of education carefully transmitted from the individual nurse to her patients, one household at a time, to produce the desired end: what she calls "a neat, well-trained consumptive."[42] Her perspective assumes that the ideal nurse is an effective teacher and that the ideal patient is a willing student with the power to effect change in his or her environment, a doubtful possibility given the rigorous discipline La Motte expected patients to exercise following the nurse's recommendations. Access to fresh air, even in the cold months of winter, resting for long periods of time, eating wholesome and nourishing food, and practicing a careful hygienic regimen to avoid the spread of the disease through sputum demanded resources, in both finances and time, which most of her patients did not possess.

In one article, La Motte includes a sketch of a model of Dr. Knopf's "window tent" on display at the American Tuberculosis Exhibition in New York City in the fall of 1908. This tent was a popular attraction because of "its extreme simplicity and excellence."[43] La Motte spends roughly a third of the article documenting the mechanism of the tent and praising its attributes. While she finds much to admire about it from the nurse's perspective, it must have been a tremendous hardship for patients to have their faces constantly exposed to frigid or humid air.

Her fascination with restoring health and order to her patients' environments through the latest innovations is also manifest in her great appreciation for the "exhibit … of Miss Damer … of the Bellevue [Hospital]."[44] The exhibit reproduced a tenement room, unclean and in a state of disarray before the nurse's arrival, alongside a "remodelled" room with "everything neat, clean, and in order, after the visits of the nurse."[45] In La Motte's vision, the individual nurse wields potentially great transformative power. She can re-order her patients' worlds, removing filth and illness through her educative efforts. La Motte does give some attention to structural issues that come into play in this remaking of the tenement. She mentions that in the "after" version of the room, there is "a window … in accordance with new tenement-house laws,"[46] acknowledging that the nurses' efforts need to work in accordance with legislation to improve the living conditions of the poor.

However, in her early writings La Motte does little more than allude to the broader economic and social issues that need to be addressed in order to eradicate the disease; instead, she expected the individual nurse's efforts to bear fruit, even advocating for coercive measures such as exploiting food to compel patients to follow the prescribed regimen. Charity agencies in Baltimore often provided milk and eggs, at the time the foods best believed to boost the weight and health of tubercular patients, to those who could not afford them. La Motte sees such charitable organizations and nurses working in conjunction so nurses can control the stream of food to needy patients. She observes that the supply of milk and eggs "renders it possible for the nurse to bring about changes in his mode of life which she could not otherwise accomplish."[47] For example, when a patient does not follow the nurse's advice regarding hygiene and access to fresh air, she might "hint that they [milk and eggs] will be withdrawn if he is not able or willing to fulfil [*sic*] his share of the compact."[48] Although admitting in this sentence that there are patients who cannot exercise sufficient control over their environments to comply with the recommendations, she does not follow up with analysis of the conditions that form the obstacle; rather, she comments blithely, "It is unfortunately true that there are numbers of patients who can only be reached by this means."[49] For La Motte, then, coercion and even actual withdrawal of nutritious food from patients whose bodies in the ideal nurse–patient relationship are of primary concern is a legitimate form of "care."

The concept of care in La Motte's writings defies the stereotype of the nurse as an "angel at the bedside," expressing her maternal instinct through careful nurturing of her patient's body and spirit. La Motte's writing makes clear that her tubercular patients were obstacles to the health of her real concern: the larger community, in this case, Baltimore. At the end of the 1905 article, she observes that with few exceptions most of the patients with tuberculosis are "doomed," yet the public should continue to have faith in the labor of the tuberculosis nurse because "the benefits of this work are not for him, but for the community."[50] Most of the tuberculosis patients were among the working poor, many of them immigrants and African Americans clustered in the slums. From La Motte's perspective, these individuals are not part of the community that needs protection but a source of contagion to be controlled and neutralized. In many ways her language regarding the working poor and African Americans mirrors that used by many reformers of the period who saw these "others" as a menace to white middle-class society.[51]

La Motte's view of the poor with whom she worked is also reflected in another kind of writing she was doing during this period that emerged from her nursing experiences. In "Humor of the Districts,"[52] La Motte mines her interactions with the urban poor for a series of sketches featuring a nurse and her patients. Published in the "Stray

Bits" section near the end of the *Johns Hopkins Nurses Alumnae Magazine* and in the "Loose Threads in a Skein" section of *Charities and the Commons*–also near the end of that week's publication–the sketches were intended to provide a bit of entertainment for readers who perhaps, like La Motte, were in need of a humorous respite from the rigors and fatigue of their professions. She explains in a prefatory remark to the first set of sketches published that:

> All of the following little stories are true and have come within the experience of the district nurse, in her rounds among the patients. These little incidents have done much to lessen the tension of difficult days and to brighten those which seemed rather too full of the sufferings of these "district people." In all cases the humor was unconscious on the part of the people themselves, and therein lies its greatest charm–the quaint and ingenious manner of thinking and feeling, which it is the nurse's privilege to come closely in contact with and to appreciate.[53]

Although La Motte claims she cherishes her relationship with the poor of "the district," the sketches themselves belie that idea; La Motte mocks her patients, imitating their accents on the page and exaggerating the informalities of their speech. African Americans appear frequently, men such as "Big Aleck," described as "a fine old negro of the old type" who is perplexed when the nurse asks his age. He responds, "'I don' know 'm, I wuz bo'n in slavery, but once when our church got afire, 'bout twenty years ago, ma age done got burnt up.'"[54] La Motte intends for his response to communicate a folksy humor, inviting the reader to laugh at the simple response of the patient. It is unsurprising that La Motte would possess the prejudices of so many of her class and race. However, given her rising status in the field and frequent participation in public conversations about public health approaches to tuberculosis, it is important to consider how her perceptions of class and race were brought to bear on her understanding of the disease and how they affected her articulation of the causes and prevention of tuberculosis.

It is evident that after "three years' experience among the poor of Baltimore" her faith in education was eroding.[55] In her 1908 presentation at the Sixth International Congress on Tuberculosis, held in Washington, DC, she essentially proclaims the failure of education as a tool to reach the vast majority of tubercular patients. Always blunt in style, she wrote her speech to provoke her audience, using stronger language than in her earlier writings to describe those she claims cannot benefit from education because "their moral as well as their physical resistance is low–a fatal combination."[56] She proclaims that "the day-laborer, the shop-girl, the drunken negro … are by nature weak, shiftless, and lacking in initiative and perseverance."[57] She clearly brings her class and race assumptions to bear in her interpretation of the behavior of the poor while simultaneously acknowledging the problem of the environment, pointing out that "the crowded quarters in which these people live mean inevitable contamination of the patient's household."[58] While considering how individuals and social conditions intersect to spread tuberculosis, she concludes that education is "a method that depends for its usefulness on the possession of certain mental and moral qualities, combined with the financial means of maintaining a certain standard of living."[59]

Because so few people have this golden combination, education, something she had spent three years promoting, was of extremely limited use. Rather than extending her analysis to examine the root problems of crowded and unsanitary living conditions, a logical target of her zeal for reform, La Motte instead advocates in the last brief paragraph of her presentation for a different approach. She suggests that "the homes of the poor should be regularly and competently inspected," and when a case of tuberculosis is detected, "the State should step in and protect the community by removing from it the source of contagion."[60] The energy of her writing and activism from this point forward is directed at highlighting the shortcomings of her earlier position, arguing for stringent forms of social control aimed at rooting out tubercular patients and putting them under the surveillance of the state in sanatoria. She again favors coercive measures, this time, those that can be implemented on a wider scale. Recognizing the failure of attempting to prevent the spread of tuberculosis through individual efforts, she begins advocating more frequently and vocally for structural changes involving local and state agencies to legitimize and legalize coercive measures, enabling health-care professionals to better control patients' diseased bodies.

Not all of her peers in the anti-tuberculosis crusade agreed with her position. As historian Jessica Robbins observes, La Motte "called for an approach that radically de-emphasized traditional nursing values of providing compassionate care for individual patients in favor of a single-minded focus on containing infection in the population as a whole."[61] This distancing of the nurse from her patient made some of La Motte's peers uneasy. Robbins traces how at the Twelfth Annual Convention of the Nurses' Associated Alumnae of the United States in Minneapolis in 1909, other responders suggested that education still had a role to play in prevention and could be used to keep patients in their homes,[62] although their protestations were often fueled by a practical recognition that there were not enough beds in institutions. Although Robbins correctly suggests that these nurses maintained their faith in education as a useful tool, some nurses were not advocating for the continued teaching of preventative measures to people in their homes; rather, they were suggesting that education be put to a larger use. Adelaide Nutting for example states that "we want better housing conditions and we want better wages for our children. When children receive this instruction they are going to demand better homes and higher wages."[63] She saw educating the next generation of reformers and advocates as one way to change the structural conditions undermining the fight against the spread of tuberculosis.

The discussion over the efficacy of education and the need to segregate patients in sanatoria continued in the *Journal of the Outdoor Life* (*JOL*), the monthly publication of the National Association for the Study and Prevention of Tuberculosis. La Motte's talk at the 1908 International Congress on Tuberculosis was printed in the April 1909 edition of *JOL*, and the presentation of Mary E. Lent, La Motte's co-author, long-time friend, and the head of the IVNA of Baltimore, appeared in the journal in September.[64] Lent's position echoes La Motte's; she proposed that many patients could not apply what they learned about preventing the spread of their disease because of a "lack of sufficient moral strength" and a "lack of the material necessities and requisite surroundings."[65] She ultimately argues that "the true function" of the nurse is to reveal to "the general public … the conditions that render futile the present efforts to eliminate the disease" and to convince patients that "removal to a comfortable and attractive hospital" is a necessary and beneficial step.[66]

Mabel Jacques, the first woman in Philadelphia to serve as a tuberculosis nurse for the Visiting Nurse Society, also presented at the International Congress. As historian Barbara Bates notes, Jacques later critiqued Lent, and La Motte implicitly, for neglecting to consider the happiness of the families she attended and advocating for the institutionalization of advanced cases, even when it meant separating family members.[67] In the November 1909 issue of *JOL*, Jacques wrote an explicit reply to Lent's position, chiding her for believing that it was possible to alter the "habits and customs of generations ... in four years."[68] She urges her to be more patient and to persist in the effort to educate patients; the payoff will be doing away with tuberculosis and "promoting happiness, that great factor of health, which cannot too often be brought to mind."[69]

Jacques' position took for granted the importance of the family and the concept of happiness, yet, in her writings about tuberculosis, La Motte never prioritized the welfare of the individual, a move that would have contradicted her insistent demand that the nurse's only object of concern was the public's health. In fact, when she discusses the parent–child relationship in her writing, she attacks the affection parents show their children, which ultimately spreads the disease through cuddling, calling it "the sheer brute affection of the ignorant and selfish."[70]

It is evident in subsequent articles that La Motte was not swayed by arguments by Jacques and others that individual rights and familial relationships needed to be safeguarded during the fight against tuberculosis; rather, in subsequent publications, she returned in full force to her articulation of the failure of education. To bolster her arguments about the dangers posed by the uneducated poor, she employed a rhetorical strategy common to reformist writings: documentary photographs. In a co-authored article, La Motte and Lent explain the role of photographs: they "are herewith reproduced in the hope that they will serve without further comment to demonstrate fully the facts which lead us to the conclusions stated above."[71] The people pictured, primarily African Americans or immigrant whites, are supposed to convey by their racial and ethnic otherness their danger to the larger community, yet the photographs reveal nothing about the subjects' supposed ignorance and inability to manage the symptoms of their disease. They are often carefully dressed, clustered in posed group shots, and face the camera, indicating their clear intention to cooperate with the photographer's wishes.

With their choice to include these kinds of photographs, Lent and La Motte aligned themselves with the work of photographer Lewis Hine. Hine was famous for his social documentary photography, particularly for his series taken for the National Child Labor Committee from 1906 to 1918. His photos were printed in *Charities and the Commons* and its successor the *Survey*, publications with which La Motte was familiar and in which her own work appeared. As a reader of these publications, she would have learned the typical characteristics of the photodocumentary essay. It is clear that she was interested in employing the form to buttress her argument regarding the need for more drastic action to curb tuberculosis.

According to historian George Dimrock, critics understand Hine's tendency to photograph his subjects, child laborers, in the forward-facing positions employed by Lent and La Motte in their article "as evidence of Hine's sensitivity toward and respect for those whom he photographed."[72] Dimrock, however, argues against this interpretation by situating the subjects of the photographs, the working poor, in relation to the photographer, a representative of the middle class. Because of this class dynamic, Dimrock asserts, "The family members look back at the camera because they have been told to do so. Their gazes remain unproblematic because they do not have the power to contest the authority and presuppositions of the man behind the camera."[73]

La Motte did not possess the authority granted middle-class males such as Hine, but she had the authority derived from her nurse's uniform–a uniform that granted her access to people's homes, where she could ask questions about their private lives and their economic situations and make recommendations about how they should change their lives to curb the disease. She was aware of the authority she and other nurses possessed in relation to their patients and she urged them to exercise it: "Authority is a term somewhat subtle in its definition–it means that hint of power, or sureness, of knowledge, which enables one to speak with a confidence which transmits itself to others, and compels them to accept one's point of view."[74]

That authority comes to bear on her patients/subjects in these photographs. In his work, Hine represented people on whose behalf he was advocating, although as Dimrock argues within a specific power dynamic. Nonetheless, the children featured in his photographs were supposed to arouse compassion and anger in viewers and to prompt them to advocate against child labor. La Motte, on the other hand, uses the images of the people on whose behalf she was theoretically advocating to arouse fear and anger against these same people. It is hard to imagine a scenario in which any of these people would have wished to cooperate had they known that their images were destined to be used as a visual representation of the menace they posed to society. Using this visual appeal La Motte and Lent vigorously argue that, "In no other instance today is the safety, well-being and happiness of thousands of the strong, intelligent and competent members of the community made to depend upon the weak, ignorant and helpless–a reversal of the proper order of things that reduces the situation to an absurdity."[75] These photographs worked to restore the proper social order, with her white middle-class contemporaries exercising forms of control over those inferior socially, racially, and economically to them.

La Motte and Lent articulate the role of the nurse in this process as follows: "to discover and bring before the public the conditions which hinder the effectiveness of her work and prove the necessity of its being supplanted by more radical measures."[76] If the nurse was an optimistic educator in La Motte's earlier formulations of her professional role in the fight against tuberculosis, she is now a mediator of social control, a representative of her class and race interests who could use her position to coerce those who threaten the rest of the community.

La Motte also explores the power of the camera in "Strawberries–Strawberries," published in the *Survey* in 1909. In this piece she fully takes on the role of investigative journalist as she documents the living conditions of migrant workers, primarily poor immigrant whites and African Americans who leave Baltimore to earn extra money during the spring strawberry harvest. La Motte's position as a tuberculosis nurse acquaints her with this annual migration of "a large number of the consumptives under her observation,"[77] but she does not trek to the country to document the conditions there or to provide care for patients. Rather, her advocacy is brought to the pages of the *Survey*, where readers can witness the conditions for themselves and then mobilize to bring about change if they are so motivated.[78] Her approach to instilling a sense of outrage in her readers is to detail the living conditions of these temporary workers. She describes huts constructed like "stable[s]"[79] where people are housed like animals in cramped and filthy conditions. Photographs of the exteriors and interiors of the huts and people clustered in groups in front of them appear on every page of the article, visually reinforcing the terrible living conditions so conducive to spreading tuberculosis.

La Motte explains that some of her white subjects objected to these photographic intrusions because they "were ashamed"; they would only allow La Motte and her unnamed companion(s) to enter after "constant urging" and "flatly refused to let them [their quarters] be photographed."[80] Although this hesitation is inconvenient to La Motte's purpose, she grudgingly admires this pride, in contrast to "colored people" who possessed "no consciousness of their demoralized living conditions. They showed us their quarters with alacrity, good-naturedly laughing at their shortcomings, and were only too glad to be photographed."[81] For La Motte, the power of the camera serves to reinforce her existing prejudices and becomes a tool to gauge the morality of her subjects.

The end of the article picks up energy as she sums up her main points of concern: highlighting the fact that the poor living conditions are encouraging the spread of tuberculosis and undermining any benefit of being outdoors in fresh air. She returns to her concern for the larger community by pointing to the danger of having consumptives pick berries that will be consumed raw by customers, potentially providing a source of contagion. She issues a familiar warning: "The welfare, therefore, not only of those who actually engage in this occupation, but also of the rest of the community demands that some method be adopted of improving the conditions."[82] The urgency to act is communicated by the final two photographs, in which groups of white pickers are assembled in larger numbers than in the previous photographs, instilling in the reader, through their sheer number, a sense of urgency to act against this menace.

La Motte's ability to advocate against tuberculosis, and for her particular solution of removing patients to sanatoria, was augmented when she joined the Baltimore Health Department in 1909. Her first report to the department dates from that year, when she submitted a report to James Bosley, the commissioner of health, detailing the work she and another nurse had done since April. Their job "was to arrange for fumigation of houses in which there had been tuberculosis, the houses having become vacant either by the death or removal of the patient."[83] In 1910, the Department expanded the tuberculosis division, and La Motte began work as the nurse in charge, overseeing the work of the fifteen special nurses whose job it was to ferret out, report, and manage tubercular patients.

La Motte's wish for a better-organized system of surveillance came to fruition with the creation of this division. In one of her last published articles about tuberculosis, she takes a more conciliatory tone than in articles published in 1908–1911. Rather than using the strong tones of a crusader, La Motte writes as a confident administrator. Although still taking the position that advanced tubercular patients should be removed from their homes, she acknowledges more thoroughly the role of social conditions in the production and control of the disease. For the first time, too, she admits that poverty does not determine the carefulness of a patient and that municipal nurses care for patients from all economic classes who exhibit varying degrees of conscientiousness in the management of their illnesses.[84]

The reason for her measured tone is perhaps that from her administrative position, she saw less of the patients and had more of a broad view of the forces at work in the spread of tuberculosis. She was writing as a voice for the municipality and focused on "those measures instituted by a city or community by which it attempts to rid itself of tuberculosis."[85] Given her new position, she was no longer as concerned with the care an individual nurse could extend to a patient; rather, she was preoccupied with creating and managing a system with which the disease and patients in its various stages could be methodically overseen. She argued for the three things a community needed to combat tuberculosis: nurses, dispensaries, and hospitals. The nurse in particular had a unique role to play as "the great go-between between the physician and the patient, the patient and the institution."[86] She emphasizes the need to hire "strong, intelligent, and well-trained women"[87] for this particular kind of nursing. They must have not only the expected medical skills but a "strong personality … to combat opposing and frequently hostile opinions, and to bring those opinions into co-operation."[88]

Toward the end of her tuberculosis nursing career, La Motte came to see the tuberculosis nurse as someone who also needed to be an effective social worker. She argued that it was a waste of money and resources to have both nurses and social workers visiting the homes of tubercular patients and that the skills of the two could be and should be combined in the person of the tuberculosis nurse. She could easily receive training through a course or field experience to supplement her medical knowledge.[89] La Motte envisioned the tuberculosis nurse becoming a highly skilled organizer who could coordinate meeting a patient's medical and social needs while working for the betterment of the community's health. In *The Tuberculosis Nurse*, she also recognizes that because of the complexities involved in working with social agencies, charities, and the medical establishment, the experienced tuberculosis nurse would be well prepared to assume executive positions in other realms,[90] drawing attention to the way she was imagining forging new professional opportunities for herself and other women both inside and outside of nursing.

La Motte was clear that the career of the tuberculosis nurse must be a short one. She believed that the demands, both physical and mental, of the job meant that it was "not good as a steady occupation."[91] Rather, she advocated for accumulating knowledge and experience and then using them as a springboard for other kinds of jobs. While working at the Health Department from 1910 to 1913, La Motte chose to exercise her organizational and executive skills outside of nursing by using her writing and speaking abilities to advocate for women's suffrage. During these three years, La Motte became increasingly engaged in the fight for the vote and entered into very public and sometimes controversial debates about granting women voting rights. Her participation in these political efforts further strengthened her already formidable skills as a writer and speaker and eventually emboldened her to untether herself from Baltimore and tuberculosis nursing. In 1913, she struck out as a "special correspondent" for the *Sun*, tasked with covering the militant tactics of London's suffragettes, a move that would mark a permanent change in her life: while she would nurse again eventually, she would not do so in Baltimore in the milieu that had been so crucial to shaping her into a powerful nurse and activist for public health.

Notes

1 Georgina Caird Ross, JHMI, Student Applications, "Notes from Interview with Ellen La Motte," July 19, 1898.
2 Karen Buhler-Wilkerson, *False Dawn: The Rise and Decline of Public Health Nursing, 1900–1930* (New York: Garland, 1989), p. 77, n. 42.
3 Janet Wilson James, "Isabel Hampton and the Professionalization of Nursing in the 1890s," in M. J. Vogel and C. Rosenberg (eds), *The Therapeutic Revolution: Essays in the Social History of American Medicine* (Philadelphia: University of Pennsylvania Press, 1979), pp. 214–215.
4 JHMI, Student Applications, "Ellen La Motte to Adelaide Nutting," September 23, 1898.
5 *Ibid.*
6 "World of Society," *Morning News* (November 26, 1898), p. 6.
7 "Social Wilmington," *Philadelphia Inquirer* (November 20, 1898), p. 11. A "P.P.C. card," from the French "pour prendre congé," was a card that announced one's absence or departure from town.
8 Ross, "Notes."
9 JHMI, Student Applications, "Ellen La Motte to Adelaide Nutting," July 28, 1898.
10 *Johns Hopkins Hospital 13th Report of the Superintendent, 1900–1901*, p. 33. See also, "Wilmington Girl Wins Honor as a Nurse," *Evening Journal* (May 25, 1901), p. 4, which specifies that she was awarded "a scholarship, and a purse of $100."
11 "The Hospital and Training School News," *Johns Hopkins Nurses Alumnae Magazine* (hereafter *JHNAM*) 1:4 (December 1902), p. 119.
12 "News Notes," *JHNAM* 3:1 (March 1904), p. 42.
13 She is listed as having an address in Florence, Italy in "Twelfth Annual Report of the Alumnae Association of the Johns Hopkins Hospital Training School for Nurses, 1903–1904," *JHNAM* 3:3 (August 1904), p. 191.
14 Fitzgerald graduated from Johns Hopkins in 1906 and eventually served as the Edith Cavell Memorial Nurse from Massachusetts with the British Expeditionary Forces. The JHMI has a student file on Fitzgerald as well as a variety of papers and diaries from her time as a nurse during World War One. Also, see Christine E. Hallett, *Nurse Writers of the Great War* (Manchester: Manchester University Press, 2016), pp. 111–117, for more information about Fitzgerald's service and writings.
15 "News Notes," *JHNAM* 3:4 (November 1904), p. 228; "Hospital and Training-School Items," *American Journal of Nursing* (hereafter *AJN*), 5:3 (December 1904), p. 215. A note from fall 1905 observes that she worked as an operating-room nurse; see *AJN* 6:1 (October 1905), p. 63.
16 "Hospital and Training-School Items," *AJN* 5:1 (October 1904), p. 69. Van Blarcom eventually went on to have a successful career in midwifery and

working to combat blindness. The JHMI has a student file on Van Blarcom that includes a short biography and materials related to her career and life.

17 "News Notes," *JHNAM* 4:3 (August 1905), p. 111; "Hospital and Training-School Items," *AJN* 6:1 (October 1905), p. 63.

18 Ellen N. La Motte, "Early Struggles with Contagion," *AJN* 1:8 (May 1901), p. 541.

19 *Ibid.*, p. 545.

20 Ellen N. La Motte, *The Tuberculosis Nurse*, History of American Nursing (1915; repr., New York: Garland Press, 1985), p. 2.

21 Ellen N. La Motte, "A Modern Italian Hospital," *AJN* 4:12 (September 1904), p. 934.

22 Buhler-Wilkerson, *False Dawn*, p. 30.

23 La Motte, "A Modern Italian Hospital," p. 937.

24 *Ibid.*, p. 938.

25 Ellen N. La Motte, "Private Nursing in Italy," *AJN* 5:2 (November 1904), p. 106.

26 *Ibid.* Italics in the original.

27 Susan B. Reverby, *Ordered to Care: The Dilemma of American Nursing, 1850–1945* (Cambridge: Cambridge University Press, 1987), p. 21.

28 Ellen N. La Motte, "Hôpital Général, Rheims," *AJN* 5:6 (March 1905), p. 368.

29 *Ibid.*, pp. 368–369.

30 Isabel Hampton Robb (1860–1910) was the first Superintendent of Nurses and Principal of the Training School at Johns Hopkins, between 1889 and 1894. Lavinia Dock (1858–1956) was Hampton's Assistant Superintendent for three years beginning in 1890. Adelaide Nutting (1858–1948) was in the first class to graduate from Johns Hopkins in 1891 and was named Superintendent after Hampton's departure in 1894. She left in 1907 to take a position at Columbia Teachers College. While Robb and Dock left before La Motte's arrival, she presumably knew their legacies at the training school and heard about their post-Hopkins endeavors through journals, conferences, and word of mouth. Two histories include discussion of their contributions: Ethel Johns and Blanche Pfefferkorn, *The Johns Hopkins Hospital School of Nursing 1889–1949* (Baltimore, MD: Johns Hopkins Press, 1954) and Mame Warren (ed.), *Our Shared Legacy: Nursing Education at Johns Hopkins, 1889–2006* (Baltimore, MD: Johns Hopkins University Press, 2006).

31 La Motte, "Private Nursing," p. 103.

32 *Ibid.*, p. 106.

33 *Ibid.*, p. 108.

34 Ellen N. La Motte, "Tuberculosis Work of the Instructive Visiting Nurse Association of Baltimore," *AJN* 6:3 (December 1905), p. 141.

35 Jessica M. Robbins, "Class Struggles in the Tubercular World: Nurses, Patients, and Physicians, 1903–1915," *Bulletin of the History of Medicine* 71:3 (1997), p. 429.

36 La Motte, "Tuberculosis Work," p. 141.
37 *Ibid.*, pp. 141, 142.
38 *Ibid.*, p. 142.
39 Buhler-Wilkerson, *False Dawn*, p. ix.
40 La Motte, "Tuberculosis Work," p. 142.
41 *Ibid.*
42 *Ibid.*, p. 145. Jessica Robbins situates La Motte in the larger debate about the limits and possibilities of education in Jessica M. Robbins, "'Barren of Results?': The Tuberculosis Nurses' Debate, 1908–1914," *Nursing History Review* 9 (2001), pp. 35–50.
43 Ellen N. La Motte, "The American Tuberculosis Exhibition," *AJN* 6:5 (February 1906), p. 307.
44 *Ibid.*, p. 310.
45 *Ibid.*
46 *Ibid.*
47 La Motte, "Tuberculosis Work," p. 143.
48 *Ibid.*
49 *Ibid.*
50 *Ibid.*, p. 147.
51 For a discussion of nativists' fears of immigrants and their threat to public health, see A. Kraut, *Silent Travelers: Germs, Genes, and the "Immigrant Menace"* (New York: Basic Books, 1994), especially pp. 78–104. For an analysis of race theory, African Americans, and tuberculosis see S. K. Roberts, Jr., *Infectious Fear: Politics, Disease, and the Health Effects of Segregation*, Studies in Social Medicine (Chapel Hill, NC: University of North Carolina Press, 2009).
52 "Humor of the Districts" appeared twice in *JHNAM*, once in 1905 and once in 1906. In 1906, *Charities and the Commons* reprinted some of the material published in the 1905 *JHNAM* in its "Loose Threads in a Skein" column.
53 Ellen N. La Motte, "Humor of the Districts," *JHNAM* 4:4 (November 1905), p. 220.
54 *Ibid.*
55 Ellen N. La Motte, "The Unteachable Consumptive," in *Transactions of the Sixth International Congress on Tuberculosis*, vol. 3 (Philadelphia: William F. Fell, 1908), p. 257.
56 *Ibid.*, p. 258.
57 *Ibid.*, pp. 257–258.
58 *Ibid.*, p. 259.
59 *Ibid.*, p. 260.
60 La Motte, "The Unteachable Consumptive," p. 260.
61 Robbins, "Barren of Results?," p. 39.
62 *Ibid.*, pp. 39–40.

63 "Report of the Twelfth Annual Convention," *AJN* 9:12 (September 1909), p. 934.
64 Lent graduated from the Johns Hopkins Training School for Nurses in 1895 and was actively involved in public health nursing, particularly from 1903 to 1916 when she was superintendent of the IVNA. The JHMI has a slim biographical file on Lent. See also her obituary: "Mary E. Lent: A Pioneer in Public Health Nursing," *JHNAM* 46:2 (April 1947), pp. 60–62. She and La Motte maintained a friendship at least until the mid-1910s, when La Motte was using Lent's address in the United States while she was abroad.
65 Mary E. Lent, "The True Function of the Tuberculosis Nurse," *Journal of the Outdoor Life* (hereafter *JOL*) 6:9 (September 1909), p. 268.
66 *Ibid.*, pp. 268–269.
67 Barbara Bates, *Bargaining for Life: A Social History of Tuberculosis, 1876–1938* (Philadelphia: University of Pennsylvania Press, 1992), p. 245.
68 Mabel Jacques, "Saving the Home," *JOL* 6:11 (November 1909), p. 324.
69 *Ibid.*
70 Ellen N. La Motte, "The Neglected Tuberculous Child," *JOL* 7:3 (March 1910), p. 67.
71 Mary E. Lent and Ellen N. La Motte, "The Present Status of Tuberculosis Work among the Poor," *Maryland Medical Journal* 52:4 (April 1909), pp. 155–157.
72 George Dimrock, "Children of the Mills: Re-Reading Lewis Hine's Child Labour Photographs," *Oxford Art Journal* 16:2 (January 1993), p. 48.
73 *Ibid.*
74 La Motte, *The Tuberculosis Nurse*, p. 18.
75 Lent and La Motte, "The Present Status," p. 154.
76 *Ibid.*, p. 157.
77 Ellen N. La Motte, "Strawberries–Strawberries," *Survey* 22:18 (July 1909), p. 632.
78 La Motte's article is cited by the *Sun* as the catalyst for an amendment to the Food Products Inspection bill. See "For New Health Laws," *Sun* (March 3, 1914), p. 7.
79 La Motte, "Strawberries," p. 633.
80 *Ibid.*, pp. 636–637.
81 *Ibid.*, p. 637.
82 *Ibid.*, p. 639.
83 Ellen N. La Motte, Baltimore City Archives, RG19, Health Department, Annual Reports, "Report of Tuberculosis Nurses' Division." *Annual Report of the Sub-Department of Health, Department of Public Safety, 1909.*
84 Ellen N. La Motte, "Municipal Care of Tuberculosis," *AJN* 12:11 (August 1912), p. 940.
85 *Ibid.*, p. 935.
86 *Ibid.*, p. 938.

87 *Ibid.*
88 *Ibid.*, p. 941.
89 Ellen La Motte, "The Nurse as Social Worker," *Visiting Nurse Quarterly* 3:4 (October 1911), p. 79.
90 La Motte, *The Tuberculosis Nurse*, p. 23.
91 La Motte, "Municipal Care," p. 941.

2

La Motte and suffrage, 1910–1913

By the end of September 1913, having left her nursing responsibilities behind her, La Motte, reporting as a special correspondent from London for the Baltimore *Sun*, published the fifth of six reports about the tactics, meetings, and trials of militant suffragettes. In it she describes standing on a London street selling copies of the *Suffragette*, the weekly journal of the WSPU:[1]

> [T]here is nothing more enlightening than paper selling. … For the opinions of those who pass by are not self-contained. On the contrary, their opinions and their antagonism are so strong and so bitter that they wreak them on the person who is quietly offering for sale a paper which stands for justice and equality.[2]

La Motte's decision to stand her ground and sell the paper despite the abuse hurled in her direction marked a continuation of her interest in and dedication to campaigning on behalf of causes concerned with political justice and the public good. The eight years, from 1905 to 1913, that she spent working as a tuberculosis nurse in Baltimore, where she developed a reputation as an expert in the field and earned a name for herself regionally, nationally, and even internationally as an anti-tuberculosis crusader, resulted in her giving frequent talks and publishing often. This rising involvement in debates about public health issues was accompanied by increased participation in the suffrage cause. She supported those efforts by drawing on the skills she had acquired through her nursing career to speak and write on behalf of votes for women and by connecting the power of the vote to the possibility of bringing about the social changes needed to eradicate tuberculosis and other public health threats while simultaneously working to increase women's political and social equality.

La Motte was actively involved with the local suffrage movement in Baltimore and was a member of the Just Government League of Maryland by early 1910. At the time, Mary E. Lent[3] was president of the organization and Florence Sabin, a 1900 graduate of the Johns Hopkins Medical School and the first woman to serve as a faculty member at the university, was the corresponding secretary.[4] Baltimore had a vibrant activist community devoted to the suffrage cause, and Johns Hopkins women were an important part of it, lending their speaking and writing skills to raise awareness of the importance of recognizing women as political equals. Intelligent, articulate, accustomed to public speaking, and familiar with organizing and advocating on behalf of health-related causes, women such as La Motte used the skills they had acquired and sharpened through nursing to advocate for change in the public sphere by fighting for women's right to vote.

The degree to which La Motte was engaged in suffrage efforts before 1910 is difficult to determine. Her decision to leave the comforts and security of her home at the age of twenty-five to attend nursing school suggests an independence of spirit that would have undoubtedly moved her to seek out other like-minded women, many of whom would have been interested in the political battle for equality. While in her early twenties, she is mentioned in association with bicycles, seen as an emancipatory technology for women in the 1890s, several times, first attending a dance at the Scranton Bicycle Club[5]–La Motte and her family went to the city often to visit her father's sister, Margaretta, who had married Henry Belin, Jr., a successful businessman and the president of E. I. du Pont de Nemours of Pennsylvania, in 1868. A few years after the dance, La Motte is noted in a social column as "often seen at her wheel" on the roads and byways of Wilmington and beyond.[6] The description of other Wilmingtonians, including La Motte's cousin Alfred I. du Pont and his first wife, Bessie Gardner du Pont, taking part in this activity, reflects the view of bicycling, particularly for women, as a new and exciting avenue to freedom and as a way to develop "a practical, capable new modern womanhood."[7] La Motte may have taken more serious steps beyond engagement with this forward-looking leisure activity to promote women's increased freedom and political rights, but if she belonged to groups that advocated for female suffrage before entering nursing school, no trace of her participation has been left behind.

Before departing for Johns Hopkins, she would, however, have been exposed at least to a variety of highly organized charitable and reform efforts in Wilmington, including those of the New Century Club, founded in 1889, whose goals were "philanthropic, and charitable, and moral and intellectual development."[8] Beginning in 1894, the club launched a series of activities designed to improve the city's cleanliness and its citizens' health,[9] efforts that later occupied La Motte's attention in Baltimore through her work as a nurse, advocate for the vote, and as a clubwoman. Several women she knew, such as young women in the du Pont, Gause, Lea, and Maull families, were members during the years she lived in Wilmington.[10] Clubs like these were common all over the country, as women turned their efforts to "municipal housekeeping," which "conferred an air of respectability upon what might otherwise have been considered unseemly public or political activity."[11]

In Baltimore in 1907, before her more vocal entrance into the fight for the vote in 1910, she joined the Social Service Club of Maryland.[12] The by-laws from 1907 stated that "the objects of the Club are the promotion of personal acquaintance, and the reading of papers and discussions of subjects that shall strengthen the unity of thought and opinion of philanthropic work in our city."[13] The membership roll included prominent professional women like Dr. Claribel Cone, Anna Herkner, and Dr. Lilian Welsh, and nurses such as Mary B. Dixon, Mary E. Lent, and Reiba Thélin Foster–the Club sometimes met at the Nurses Home at 1123 Madison Ave.[14] Given the involvement of prominent citizens in the fields of health care and social reform, it is not surprising that the minutes of the September meeting of 1907 show that the Executive Committee, which included La Motte's good friend and colleague, Lent, decided to develop a program of speakers for the coming year drawn from these fields. For example, Drs. Henry M. Hurd and William H. Welch were invited to speak on "Hygiene and Its Social Relations" and Julia C. Lathrop was noted as a speaker in October.[15] The club, as recorded in the minutes of its October 1907 meeting, determined that "a Committee of five be appointed to look after all legislation of interest to the Club introduced in the

City Council, and, in conjunction with the Executive Committee, to take action on the same."[16] This plan suggests that the Club wanted to do more than educate its members and promote social interaction. However, at its January 1908 meeting, a request from the United Settlements Association, "asking whether the Social Service Club would take the initiative or would join with a committee of the United Settlements Association in an attempt to secure the re-organization of the Society for the Protection of Children for the purpose of making that society the agency for the enforcement of laws and ordinances designed for the protection of child life," provoked a discussion of the question "shall the purpose of the Social Service Club be strictly educational, or shall it be also militant, assuming certain definite lines of work from time to time?"[17] The January meeting resolved that "the Executive Committee be constituted a permanent Committee on Law and Legislation, whose duty it shall be to express the views of the Club before the Legislature or City Council," thereby concluding that the Club would indeed take "militant" action when appropriate.[18]

While the minutes do not reflect which members were in attendance at various meetings, La Motte was a steady participant in club activities after she was elected secretary at the May 1908 meeting. In her first recorded minutes from an October 1908 meeting of the Executive Committee–the Club did not meet during the summer months–she noted that plans for the Club's winter program included "an evening devoted to the question of Equal Suffrage, with possible [*sic*] Jane Addams as a speaker."[19] That idea did not materialize, as evidenced in the December 1908 minutes, which document the Club's plans to finalize their speakers for the year, none of whom were going to speak about suffrage. There are many possible reasons Addams might not have been able to arrange a visit, but it is impossible that other suffrage speakers could not have been found in her stead. Presumably, the Social Service Club felt disinclined to provide a venue for exploring the issue of women's political rights. In February, the Club did agree to make available a petition from the Equal Suffrage League of Maryland that was going to be sent to Congress to request "that women be given the right to vote."[20] The petition was "to be laid on the table, to be signed after the meeting by all who wished to do so."[21] This delicate and passive approach to integrating the discussion of suffrage into the Club's activities stands in contrast to the active approach described in the next paragraph of the minutes, in which the President of the Club, Mr. Magruder, urged Club members to write to their "Maryland senators and Congressmen to support" a pending bill about the formation of the Federal Children's Bureau.[22] While La Motte only records the discussion in the objective language expected in the official Club record, given her commitment to women's rights, this lack of direct action on the subject must have been frustrating for her.

While the Club provided a way for women like La Motte to increase their education on pressing social issues and offered them an opportunity to learn to speak effectively before the city council or state legislature, club members saw their mission–as discussed after the Executive Committee rejected La Motte's suggestion to include in their program of speakers an expert on "Hook Worm disease"–as being to promote "topics of more vital interest to the social workers of Baltimore."[23] Though enfranchising women would have lent tremendous political clout to the aims of the Social Services Club, the membership was not willing to engage in the controversies around the issue lest they divert their attention–whether with hookworm or suffrage–from their goal of educating social workers. This issue became more pressing at the December 1909 meeting, when the revision of the city charter was under discussion. After members listened to a lecture about forming charters based on the unique needs of each city, Lent, identified in her role as "President of the Just Government League, spoke of the desirability of having qualified woman suffrage incorporated into the revised charter."[24] Her suggestion was supported by Mrs. J. William Funck, President of the Baltimore City Suffrage Club, and the President of the Second Branch City Council, Mr. Numsen. However, the most influential person noted, Dr. William Welch, the "President of the Charter Revision Committee, said that extension of the suffrage had nothing to do with the questions under consideration, viz. remodeling of the charter of Baltimore."[25] La Motte perfunctorily recorded: "After discussions of various kinds, the meeting adjourned."[26] Regrettably, nothing specific was said about her reaction or that of the other suffragists in the room though it must have seemed beyond disingenuous for Welch to refuse to acknowledge the importance of writing female suffrage into the city's revised charter. The question remained dormant for the rest of La Motte's turn as secretary for the 1910–1911 year as the

Club continued to engage vigorously with a variety of "municipal housekeeping" issues.

La Motte maintained her ties with the Club–she was elected treasurer again for the 1910–1911 year and provided entertainment in the way of "vaudeville sketches" during the Club's annual outing in August[27]–but her ardent wish to gain the vote could not be translated into activism in this venue and she sought out other opportunities to campaign vocally for the vote. Through the end of 1909, her focus was on publishing about and giving talks on tuberculosis and public health-related topics for a variety of audiences. Perhaps the nursing community was not quite ready to embrace the vote as a mechanism for improving social hygiene. At the Eleventh Annual Convention of the Nurses' Associated Alumnae held in May 1908, the nurses rejected a request from Anna Howard Shaw to support the following resolution:

> WHEREAS, The thinking women of America are striving more earnestly than ever before to be a helpful part of the people, in the firm belief that men and women together compose a democracy, and that until men and women have equal political rights they cannot do their best work, therefore be it
>
> *Resolved*, That the Nurses Associated Alumnae of the United States numbering 14,000 members, as a company of patriotic workers, heartily endorse every well-directed movement which tends to emancipate the women of our land and give them their rightful place in government.[28]

The minutes blandly report, "after some discussion the motion lost by a large majority."[29]

Yet, the suffrage community in Baltimore began to pick up steam in 1909, with Johns Hopkins-trained nurses and doctors a part of it. In January of that year the Equal Suffrage League held its first meeting. A Miss Hamilton gave an overview of suffrage in Baltimore, explaining

> this league makes its debut tonight. Two months ago its organizers awakened to the fact that the question of equal suffrage for men and women is one of world-wide interest and importance. There was in it, they felt, something to arrest the attention of even the most indifferent; that women independent of each other the world over were demanding suffrage. They felt this was a movement that must not be ignored and so this league was formed.[30]

Later in the year, as part of her 1909 visit to the United States, Emmeline Pankhurst gave a speech in Baltimore that may have contributed to the growing interest in the campaign. According to the coverage in the *Sun*, in contrast to the upset in Great Britain caused by Pankhurst's organization, "the agitation in the United States has been marked by no turbulence, and our suffragists have been content to conduct their campaign decorously and with due deference to the judgment of enlightened and discriminating public opinion."[31] The writer of the column remarked about the women of Baltimore in particular that "the fair sex … is not crying out for the ballot. Most of our women have no ambition to rush to the polls. They dominate domestic politics and household legislation, and that is all they desire."[32] While it is impossible to document how women like La Motte reacted on a personal level to these kinds of patronizing assessments of their political aspirations, their actions speak for them. They began organizing and advocating for the vote with renewed energy, speaking, writing, and marching with increasing frequency in hopes of pressuring legislators to take action on their demands, and in late 1909/early 1910 the Just Government League of Maryland was formed for "professional women, nurses, teachers, and business women"[33] and was to be a complement to the more conservative views of the Equal Suffrage League whose members tended to be women who did not work and were free to meet during the day whereas their professional counterparts had to arrange meetings after their work hours were done.[34]

True to its belief that "existing local conditions" do not "justify any but a conservative attitude," the Equal Suffrage League as a sponsoring body did not support the visit of Emmeline Pankhurst to Baltimore because of "her radical attitude and measures on the suffrage question."[35] In contrast, or protest more likely, the Equal Suffrage League did sponsor a visit from Ethel Snowden, an ardent English suffragist who was a critic of the Pankhursts' militant tactics, and La Motte was a member of the platform during her November 27 speech.[36] Notwithstanding some debate amongst local suffragists about the varied approaches of English suffrage campaigners, their visits were galvanizing forces: during the winter of 1909/1910 several large meetings devoted to recruiting supporters for the cause took place, and La Motte and Lent are mentioned in relation to many of them. In December 1909, Lent was elected president of the Wage Earners' Equal Suffrage League.[37] In January 1910, La Motte was a lecturer at a meeting of the Equal Suffrage League, which was convening to discuss a proposal it was bringing to the Maryland Legislature to allow women the right to vote in Baltimore.[38] Lent and La Motte's colleagues were also becoming more enthusiastic about the vote: at the seventh annual meeting of the Maryland State Association of Graduate Nurses many women pledged to join forces to support the bill being brought before the legislature through the efforts of the Equal Suffrage League and the Just Government League.[39] On February 16, 1910, hundreds of supporters went to the capital, where they presented the Woman's Municipal Suffrage Bill before the Committee on Elections.[40] Key speakers were allowed ten minutes each in which to make their pitches. Many of the appeals evoked women's traditional roles and qualities, such as Julia Rogers' assertion that "we do not wish to 'agitate'–we are Southern women … and many of us tremble at the sound of our own voices in public."[41] Lent and La Motte, women who undoubtedly did not "tremble at the sound of [their] own voices," given their extensive experience with public speaking and writing in published venues, also spoke. Lent wisely made an appeal to the sensibilities of her audience toward nurses, stating "you men all know nurses, and I think you all like us," a statement that, according to the columnist, "established a cordial entente" as she began making her argument for why working women needed the vote.[42] La Motte too spoke before the committee, bringing her knowledge of tuberculosis to the fore in a speech titled "Tuberculosis and Improved Sanitation."[43] Her brief speech "brought down the house when she lifted her lapel and revealed the police badge underneath," while arguing for the value of the nurses' work by stating, "You need our service. You value our ability. You trust our judgment, especially in this matter of giving us police authority … Yet we can't vote. Isn't that an absurd position for women like ourselves to be placed in?"[44] Notwithstanding this well-organized and well-supported effort–the petitioners brought more than 173,000 signatures to the committee–the bill was tabled and no action taken.[45]

La Motte maintained her busy schedule of campaigning while also working at the Health Department, her speaking schedule now filled by engagements on behalf of suffrage, the anti-tuberculosis campaign, and when possible, combining the two to put forth arguments for why the vote would help to solve the tuberculosis problem. She augmented her efforts beyond speaking when she served as an election observer in September of 1910, going to a polling station at 1101 Pennsylvania Avenue in the Thirteenth Precinct in the Seventeenth Ward, where for "the first time in the history of Maryland … any woman … acted in any official capacity at any election, primary or general."[46] She also used her writing skills, developed through her history of publishing on nursing-related topics, on behalf of the cause by writing for the *New Voter: A State Periodical of Fundamental Democracy and a Narrative of the Evolution of Woman Suffrage*, published by the Equal Suffrage League of Baltimore. Its prospectus stated that its "policy … is not only to be strictly impartial, but to welcome and encourage discussion on controversial points."[47] It was launched on November 15, 1910, with one of La Motte's Johns Hopkins acquaintances, Mary Bartlett Dixon, a 1903 graduate of the Johns Hopkins Training School,[48] its assistant editor. Any "club which guarantees 25 subscribers will have the right to appear as Associate Editor";[49] consequently, several suffrage organizations, including the Just Franchise League of Talbot County, the Political Equality League of Baltimore County, and the Just Government League of Maryland, had representatives on the advisory and editorial boards of the *New Voter*, with La Motte representing the Just Government League.

The purpose of the publication was articulated by Elizabeth King Ellicott, a wealthy suffragist[50] who lent financial support to the cause, in the first edition:

> *The New Voter* is a State periodical to be published in the interests of the women of Maryland to promote the enfranchisement of women in this State, and to give the latest suffrage news throughout the world. … *The New Voter* stands for active suffrage propaganda in Maryland, and for civic education of women as potential and intelligent voters … and hopes to be a bond of union and strength among all women, realizing that the status of women rests on all who feel their universal sisterhood.[51]

The writers and editors wished to promote work being done at the local and state levels but tied that activity to the national and international movements. The second piece in the first number, "The Undercurrent of the Woman's Movement," underscored that the movement "is not confined to an isolated community, but has been undertaken simultaneously in all parts of the world, thereby emphasizing the fact that it is lifted beyond a temporary and withheld privilege, and becomes an evolutionary force that molds races and makes history–becomes a part of the long conflict for human liberty."[52] The journal further linked the local struggle in Maryland to larger international currents by noting where other suffrage papers were being published around the world and reporting on news from suffrage activity in Turkey, England, Ireland, and Australia. A variety of national activities were also shared–news about bills enfranchising women that were before voters of states like South Dakota must have been encouraging to Maryland women struggling to enact similar legislation.

A third section of the journal covered the activities of "City and County Leagues of Maryland," many of which, populated by white middle-class women, conceptualized the suffrage movement as a way to empower women of their class and race to make changes in society through "social housecleaning."[53] For example, in the first issue Mayor Mahool of Baltimore is praised "because he is a good housekeeper he is a suffragist, and thinks women's votes will be of practical assistance in keeping the city clean."[54] Embracing a non-threatening role as defenders of the city's moral, social, and literal hygiene, the suffragists made no radical challenges to the way race and class affected women's lives, promoting instead their own middle-class reformist concerns and objectives for society.[55] Many of the ten issues published over the next seven months promoted education on municipal issues and how municipal government worked, often with the goal of putting forward bills in favor of "municipal suffrage for properly qualified women,"[56] such as one supported by the Just Franchise League of Talbot County. One column reported that as a result of "a gratifying increase in the desire of women for a more definite knowledge of the principles of municipal government … a course of lectures whereby they may more clearly understand these underlying principles" was being sponsored by the Equal Suffrage League at the Arundel Club, a place where clubwomen met and suffrage-related activities often took place. Similar kinds of lectures were frequently referred to in the pages of the journal, highlighting the view promoted by the editors "that government now has as much to do with social and domestic conditions as it has with business, bullets and battleships and that because this is true it is impossible for the government to reach the wisest decisions unless their decisions are based on both men's and women's opinions."[57]

Women's value, as articulated in the pages of the journal, in large part came from their capacity as mothers. One column covering "the first annual meeting of the National Association for Study and Prevention of Infant Mortality" connected the high infant mortality rate to poor housing, insufficient access to clean and safe food and water, and "lack of provision for the training of girls and women for motherhood."[58] The article inquires, "how many States and cities which make large appropriations for technical schools for boys devote equally large sums out of the public treasury for technical schools of continuation classes for girls, where they may be trained for the business of home keeping and child rearing?"[59] One way to keep fears about granting women the vote was to assure readers that women and their male allies did not wish to alter the fundamental roles of men and women; rather, the vote would strengthen women's abilities as mothers, thereby improving the lives of their children and husbands. One editorial–"Suffrage for Men"–discussed at length the benefits of the vote to men, first pointing out the shortcomings of women: their propensity for being "shrewd and underhand" as well as their tendency to be jealous of "any person or thing interfering with [marriage]" since it is "woman's *one* job."[60] The remedy for these weaknesses was the vote, which would give men "the pleasure of being able to discuss with … someone as bright and interested as themselves."[61] The writer urged women to "try and overcome your reputation for fighting against men; don't antagonize them, don't look down on them … get them somehow to 'eat from your hand.' Then you can inoculate the food against the 'ancient received opinions.' "[62]

The arguments laid out in the column echo those of essayist Mary Wollstonecraft from more than a century earlier about the importance of educating women to become better partners to their husbands. In lamenting the way women were poorly educated and "degraded by mistaken notions of female excellence," which "produces a propensity to tyrannize, and gives birth to cunning, the natural opponent of strength, which leads them to play off those contemptible infantile airs that undermine esteem even whilst they excite desire,"[63] Wollstonecraft asks, "Can they govern a family, or take care of the poor babes whom they bring into the world?"[64] Her cry that women need opportunities to become better educated to fulfill their functions as wives and mothers, one hundred years later, evolved into a demand for the vote for the same reason. Both Wollstonecraft and the suffragists embraced positions that, while they may have been threatening to traditionalists, ultimately aimed to maintain the power and authority of men and the separate domains of women.

With regard to other topics, such as race, the columns of the *New Voter* also took a conservative position. The writers for the paper did not attempt to mobilize African American women to campaign for the vote. Unsurprisingly, the journal was generally silent on the issue of the status of African Americans in relation to political power in Maryland.[65] One columnist, advocating for the "centralization" of suffrage efforts in Maryland and identifying problems in mobilizing as a cohesive force, remarked "the State is small, and made smaller by the black belt."[66] The dismissive line suggests that the black population had to be subtracted from the overall population before a plan could be formulated to unite the presumably white groups lobbying for different voting measures for women. Other than this brief mention of African Americans, they are virtually absent from the pages of the *New Voter*, and other marginalized groups, such as immigrants, are referred to as objects of derision, such as when one writer argues that women should not be perceived as inferior to "the degraded foreigner who swarms our shores."[67] Another writer saw the advantage of giving women the vote, because "when women vote they will have the power to decrease the supply of women workers by assisting in the regulation of immigration laws."[68]

La Motte's views, as expressed in the pages of the *New Voter*, regarding the purpose of the vote, gender, and race were more nuanced. The sketches she published mocking African American patients reflect racist attitudes,[69] yet, like many progressives, she held contradictory attitudes about race and class and understood the need to make changes at the structural level to create a more just society. While many of her colleagues writing for the paper saw the vote as a "cure" for social ills, La Motte also talked about it explicitly as a mode of prevention: women endowed with the vote would help to create a more just and safe society. In October 1910, she gave a speech to the Men's Guild of Garrett Park Episcopal Church in which her primary purpose was to make a case for why women needed a political voice to combat the corruption of judges in Baltimore city courts. She attested that, having frequently attended trials, "when a man is accused of having wronged a young girl almost invariably he is acquitted or else the punishment inflicted is very slight."[70] She brought her awareness of the way gender affected justice to her column, "Court Proceedings," later titled "Justice," initiated in the second issue of the *New Voter*. Its stated purpose was "to review, issue by issue, all cases of a certain class that come up for trial in the Criminal Courts of our city."[71] It appeared in seven of the ten issues of the *New Voter*, and while La Motte appears to be the author of most of them, some of the columns may have been the result of a collaborative effort. Ellicott chaired a committee that attended trials of the kind discussed in the column;[72] one woman kept track of decisions, presumably La Motte, who then used the material for the column, though Lola Carson Trax, a contributing editor representing the Just Franchise League of Talbot County, may have aided in writing, or have written, at least the final column.[73]

The first column sets out its purpose and analyzes the law and its evolution, explaining that "through the enactment and enforcement of laws, society attempts to protect itself from individuals or from conditions which threaten its welfare. Law, therefore, is an expression of public opinion concerning public welfare."[74] In contrast to the idea that laws intend to protect the public good, she writes:

> [W]e may find upon the statute books laws which are not the expression of the will of the whole people, but which are merely the expression of the will of a certain group or class of people. Such legislation is called class legislation. Such laws are unjust, in that they are created by a privileged class, and designed to benefit and protect that class, at the expense of another class of people against whom they discriminate.[75]

La Motte further explains that her interest in the law and justice emerges "not … so much with the punishment of the criminal as with the protection of the community."[76] This position echoes that expressed in the summation of her work in the tuberculosis field, *The Tuberculosis Nurse*, in which she unequivocally argues that "nurses … fail to recognize the real issue, and think that it is the actual care of the patient which is the thing to be considered. This is totally wrong– *we work through the patient to gain our ends, but he himself is not the main object.*"[77] From her perspective, the patient is only a means of ensuring the health of the community. In the case of the courts, she asserts that safeguarding the community can be carried out by examining one class of crimes in particular: those in which "the aggressor is always a man and the victim is always a woman or child."[78] Bringing the gross injustice of men receiving light or no prison terms even when found guilty to the attention of the reading public formed a call to activism to create more equitable courts.

At the heart of the issue is that "a woman's life is a cheap thing. Her honor and happiness are cheap things. So say our laws."[79] When women are "betrayed, the man who betrays her is either acquitted or else given a trifling few months in jail; if she has a child by him, the father is required to pay seven dollars a year for seven years, and then his duty to it is done."[80] Because of the focus on the result of charges brought against those harming women and children, the cases discussed often involved "bastardy" and "Carnal Knowledge" with the male offenders receiving light sentences or no sentences at all. She highlights the absurdity of a professed criminal being declared not guilty, such as in the case of "Geo. Proper … accused of selling liquor to minors. He confessed to being guilty. Verdict rendered, *not guilty*."[81] In one particularly egregious case, a man, Miller, "was accused of having ruined his step-daughter, a girl of 14."[82] Having raped her, he tried to "produce a criminal abortion" after discovering her pregnancy.[83] Despite testimony on the part of the girl and her mother, which provided "conclusive evidence," the jury found him not guilty because "the dreadful facts" convinced the jury that Miller might receive a "heavy sentence."[84] To avoid this possibility and "to save the prisoner," they found him not guilty.[85] Not satisfied with merely recording the outrageous facts of cases and sentences, the final column, possibly authored or co-authored by Trax, tried to follow up on the aftermath of assault by interviewing the mother of minors who ranged from "10 to 16" and were attacked by men from "25 to 72."[86] The cases include multiple men attacking a girl of fifteen and infecting her with sexually transmitted diseases yet receiving only a fine of five dollars each. The parents of these girls, "regardless of color or nationality," felt "a despairing hopeless, heart rending acceptance, or an indignant rebellion against the injustice."[87] The final column ends on a powerful note, stating "each particular case is a protest against lack of protective legislation for young girls, and the leniency of men officials in dealing with men offenders. A contemplation of this one phase of public work should make all people believe in woman suffrage."[88]

The column lacks the same force when addressing racial inequality. La Motte did question the role of race while examining gender inequality in sentencing to a limited degree. Given her declared intention to examine cases of "class legislation," reflecting on how white juries and judges dealt differently with African Americans could certainly form part of her project, and she did some limited exploration of the issue when she described several cases in the December 1910 column, in which she documents several white men being treated with a light hand. In contrast, several African American men received stiffer sentences than those typically awarded for "felonious assault."[89] The explanation, she writes, is that

> during these last two weeks three negroes have been brought to trial on the charge of Carnal Knowledge. In order to secure a conviction, these charges were changed to Felonious Assault. Convictions were obtained. [H]owever, in each case, and in two instances the sentences given were fairly long ones, in this way assuring protection to the community. The charges against these men were pressed to a finish. The cases were neither *stet.* nor acquitted. *But* these men were negroes. Let us see how it fares when a white man is accused of a similar charge.[90]

The issue of race was not returned to in subsequent columns, and it is easy to imagine that La Motte was not encouraged or particularly motivated to continue exploring the similar ways in which those in power, white men, were bringing their prejudices to bear on the sentences doled out in the supposedly neutral territory of the court.

Her column came to an end with the final issue of the *New Voter*. Though the editorial staff announced their intention to resume publication "when the leaves begin to color and fall" and "to come back and send you a paper full of enthusiasm and hope,"[91] they did not publish again, as the Board of Directors later explained, "in order to concentrate our efforts … and to publish a monthly bulletin of local plans and results."[92] La Motte took the summer of 1911 to travel to Europe with Lent, who was recovering from an unnamed illness, where they spent almost five months, mostly in Switzerland,[93] before returning to Baltimore in September. While La Motte did not have the *New Voter* to occupy her few free hours outside of nursing, the fall of 1911 was a busy time for La Motte personally. After her return, she began corresponding with "Louise."[94] The identity of "Louise" remains unknown, but it is possible that she is Louise Carey Rosett, to whom La Motte left $5,000 in her will.[95] Rosett was born on February 2, 1887 to Francis King Carey, a prominent lawyer and businessman in Baltimore, and Anne Galbraith, who started the Gilman Country School for Boys and was involved in philanthropic efforts in the city.[96] Rosett made her debut in the winter of 1905[97] and later attended Bryn Mawr, where her cousin, M. Carey Thomas, was serving as President.[98] Like other members of her wealthy and socially engaged family, she developed interests in fighting for the public good through campaigning for workers' rights and the vote for women. Her debut speech in favor of women's suffrage, made at the Locust Point settlement house in May of 1910, promoted woman suffrage as a mechanism to improve the lives of working women, suggesting "that unions would be a big help to women, and that true democracy meant equal chances for both sexes."[99] In December 1910, she volunteered for the Junior Suffrage League, which did support work for the Equal Suffrage League and the Just Government League.[100] In conjunction with La Motte, at a meeting of the Just Government League in January of 1911, she opposed Edith Houghton Hooker's proposal to adopt a regular platform.[101] La Motte is described as having fought " 'tooth and nail' and with arguments which for the moment were close to unanswerable."[102] La Motte objected to Hooker's platform because she felt "that certain legislation which it advocated might be passed by the male voters or through efforts of the 'antis,' which, in effect, would 'spike the suffragists' guns.' "[103] Hooker's position that the league needed to embrace "definite principles, thus giving an argument for the right of women to vote"[104] won the day and the Just Government League adopted her nine planks, many of which focus on improving the lives of women and protecting and supporting children, especially girls.

Through their joint work on behalf of the Just Government League, Rosett and La Motte had an acquaintanceship at least and potentially a more complex connection. The "Louise" of the letters was someone with whom La Motte had a relationship at least in the spring of 1911, as she describes in a letter to a friend, Amy Wesselhoeft von Erdberg. "Louise" resumed writing to La Motte after La Motte's return to Baltimore in September and La Motte concluded that she "was thoroughly satisfied with her independence, with having broken away from her conventional surroundings, and with her place that she was making for herself, and with her work."[105] Rosett had been working in New York City on behalf of female workers since the summer of 1911,[106] and in the fall, she made a decision to relocate permanently to

New York City.[107] La Motte's relationship with "Louise" came to a head in December, when "Louise" went to visit her in her office and they went "over the whole frightful business," which concluded with La Motte deciding to end things because "she has her family and sisters to consider" whereas La Motte "was ready to go with her–anywhere–to give up my work and all here, and together we could find work and freedom beyond the reach of any one."[108] "Louise" refused her poignant entreaty, though La Motte declared that she could leave her work "with a clear mind, feeling that I had made my contribution to society."[109] At this point La Motte did not believe that "Louise" was acting out of fear; rather, her concern for her "people" prevented her from taking the leap of going away with La Motte and being condemned for having a lesbian relationship. As La Motte put it in her typically pithy way: "Traditions of caste are strong."[110]

Though La Motte purported to be content with the knowledge that "she loves me very dearly … I have given her back her faith in human nature … and I was the only person she has ever cared for in her curious abnormal life,"[111] in the next section of the letter she asks her friend plaintively, "where's the justice …? All I know is, I'm unhappy and it all hurts so."[112] The missive ends with her expressing her gratitude to Wesselhoeft von Erdberg when she asks her, "Do you know, whatever I am, I owe entirely to my friends? I seem to be a weak but compound sort of copy of them."[113] Yet, La Motte's belief that she and "Louise" had resolved the question of whether they could pursue a romantic relationship was not long lived. As she explains in a follow-up letter to Wesselhoeft von Erdberg written four days later, she contacted "Louise" because she "could not stand it any longer. I felt I was betraying a trust–I could not feel honest nor satisfied with the last decision we had come to."[114] Needing to adhere to her authentic desire for "Louise" that could not be quelled by deferring to social expectations, she asked to see her again. At their meeting, La Motte used "every argument I could think of" to persuade "Louise" to tell her family about their relationship and to go away with her abroad.[115] Clearly, La Motte did not intend to leave her life quietly had "Louise" accepted her proposal; she wanted them to go forward honestly, leaving jobs and families with the news of their relationship. "Louise," however, could only repeat how much she loved La Motte and explain that "she could not give up social position and family pride," that her sisters could not marry men of "position" if these men knew of her.[116] La Motte once again abandoned her attempts to bring "Louise" around to embracing their love for each other and accepting the censure and rejection that would accompany that decision. She could only conclude: "it was ingrained, inborn, inbred, and that there was no use in trying to help her."[117]

La Motte positions "Louise's" refusal, rejection really, as a refusal of help to find her way to an honest life. La Motte claims that in regards to her own feelings, "I feel singularly free, Amy. I haven't dragged my standard in the mud–I've done my best to live up to principles I believe in–to live up to them, no matter what it might cost. My soul is free and honest and I have nothing whatever to regret."[118] La Motte was determined to adhere to her principles that, though undefined in this letter, emerged from a need to live honestly and without fear of censure. She cannot, however, have been honest about her sexuality in a public way or her position in Baltimore and at the Health Department would have been imperiled. Apparently for her, the willingness to throw away her profession and social circle, even if she did not actually have to do so, was proof enough that she had the strength to live in defiance of society's expectations. "Louise" could not take that plunge so La Motte tried to dismiss the affair by explaining, "I have discharged my responsibility towards that child … Now catch me trying to develop souls in the daughters of the idle rich. Good Lord."[119] Yet, she continued her description of her own freedom and reasons for her actions for another paragraph before commenting, "My poor little Louise–my poor little child–I don't in the least mind sharing her suffering with her, if it gets any where–but just as a dead-end occupation–I can't see the reason of that."[120] La Motte's reference to "Louise" as a "child" several times in the letters suggests she was younger than La Motte–Rosett was fifteen years her junior–and someone who needed her tutoring to navigate her way to a fulfilled life.

"Louise" having definitively refused La Motte's support, love, and mentoring, La Motte had no choice but to move on from the sadness she experienced as a result of this break. By March 1912, she had regained her equilibrium and once again wrote to Wesselhoeft von Erdberg, devoting only one paragraph to "L" to communicate that "on a terrible pinnacle of virtue, not wishing to bring disgrace and unhappiness on her family, or risk their ever hearing of the thing which might have troubled them. She has gone straight into another affair, again with a married man, and from what I hear, to the limit."[121] Apparently, an affair with a married man was a scandal "Louise" saw as acceptable to her family in contrast to the shame a lesbian relationship would bring. Rosett was to bring unwanted attention and scandal to her family when she took up with Joshua Rosett, "a playwright, a Socialist, and a physician," originally from Vitebsk in what is now Belarus.[122] He divorced his first wife in August 1912 and by December 1913 he and Louise Carey were engaged,[123] an announcement that caused a sensation in Baltimore when the Jewish socialist doctor was to be connected through marriage to the patrician Carey family.[124]

The emotional tumult La Motte experienced during this period did not interfere with her nursing work and campaigning for suffrage and related causes.[125] As she wrote to Wesselhoeft von Erdberg in March 1912, she and her colleagues had "been having a very very busy winter of it, and have been going hard all the time" in pursuit of the planks outlined by Hooker in January 1911.[126] They were trying to get a bill passed limiting the women's working day to ten hours, as well as other child labor, compulsory education, and anti-saloon bills, while writing a new charter, presumably for the Just Government League. She also discussed two suffrage bills, one of which was "defeated promptly" while the other was "still in committee," but since it was "for municipal suffrage only" it was "suffrage with the fangs drawn, since it admits taxpaying women only."[127] One of the bill's key authors, Elizabeth King Ellicott, defended the bill as a "practical test of equal suffrage by presenting bills which will crystallize public opinion and make a living issue of this national question reduced to its simplest and most obvious terms."[128] Ellicott thanked women like La Motte who owned no property so would not benefit from the passage of her proposed bill for supporting it and La Motte herself wrote in favor, despite reaping no benefits from this new legislation, commenting that "Even the most conservative will admit that women who are taxed for the up-keep of the government ought to have some say as to what becomes of their money and what sort of men shall administer the government they help to support."[129] Putting the interest of the group ahead of individual benefits, she ended her statement by observing, "And those of us who are merely onlookers, see in this enfranchisement of a certain few women, the first step towards the break down called sex disqualification which has hampered us through the ages."[130] In her letter to Wesselhoeft von Erdberg she again rationalized the bill's limited scope by commenting that it "was but an entering wedge" that probably was "doomed" to fail.[131]

La Motte was in fact correct: it did fail. Supporters had banded together, as the Just Government League and the Equal Suffrage League had in 1910, to present a bill to the Committee on Constitutional Amendments in early 1912. Members of the Just Government League of Maryland, the Equal Suffrage League, the Maryland State Woman Suffrage Association, the Men's League for Woman Suffrage, and the College Equal Suffrage League traveled to Annapolis en masse to give speeches, including one by Lent, to draw attention to the bill.[132] Despite this united effort the bill did not receive committee support and was voted down when it was presented to the House of Delegates the next month, the delegates making familiar and patronizing arguments about how "woman … should be permitted to remain the pure, loving, noble gentle creature that she is."[133] Voting would potentially make women enter into public life more frequently, resulting in their going to "barrooms and similar resorts" where they would be coarsened by exposure to "insults" by men.[134] Mr. William T. Warburton, "Republican floor leader," even gave as an example of this coarsening an incident in which the President of the Just Government League refused to shake his hand because she judged him "a coward."[135] Women like Lent and La Motte were undoubtedly familiar with the way the femininity of politically engaged women was called into question, particularly that of childless working women like them. One delegate even suggested that the logical explanation for why a woman would have the time and interest to attend a legislative hearing had to be because she did not have children.

The women were accustomed to having their feminine identities questioned and their professionalism as nurses doubted because of their political activities. After their February 1910 trip to Annapolis to campaign for the vote, La Motte and Lent came under fire in an anonymous letter to the editor of the *Sun* that sarcastically noted that "the superintendent of the Instructive Visiting Nurses' Association and the chief of the city tuberculosis nurses have apparently found their professional duties so light that they are able to devote their entire time to the hustings and the holding of political meetings."[136] The writer mockingly concludes that "the white plague has been stamped out and that the indigent sick no longer need looking after, which is certainly a glorious consummation."[137] As a final blow the letter ends with the suggestion that "no further contributions from the benevolent are needed for the fight against tuberculosis if the battle has already been fought and won and the victors rest on their laurels."[138] The suggestion that they were neglecting their duties in favor of political agitation must not have sat well with La Motte and Lent given their years-long commitment to their public health nursing work. One of their champions took umbrage at the portrayal of the women and defended their "professional ability and experience" and the time they gave, Lent in particular, to aiding with "words of help and encouragement to some mothers and teachers who deal with many perplexing problems that arise as to the welfare of the children" at the Locus Point settlement.[139]

The following year, when the Instructive District Nursing Association of Boston (IDNA) was looking to hire a nurse to take charge of the organization, Ellen Phillips Crandall, after turning down the job, highly recommended that Katharine B. Codman, the president of the organization, hire La Motte, explaining that she "is well educated, writes ably and speaks with ease and force."[140] The subsequent exchange of letters between Codman and those writing in reference to La Motte's training, experience, and personality offers rare insight into La Motte's skills, complex personality, and how her political activities were perceived as affecting her nursing. Although Crandall admired La Motte's ability to speak forcefully, other writers, especially the society women involved with public health nursing and reform efforts, such as Elizabeth King Ellicott, were more hesitant about her strong personality even as they praised her nursing and executive skills. Ellicott had known La Motte for a number of years through suffrage work, including on the *New Voter*, and had been in Baltimore while La Motte built her reputation as a tuberculosis expert. She claimed that "Miss La Motte is a personal friend of mine & I consider her one of the ablest women in the nursing profession," and assured Mrs. Codman that "her executive ability is unusual– her power of taking hold of new & hard problems, her quickness of mind & her ability to reach new conclusions, & to see dangerous or promising tendencies which affect the progress of work are joined to a power of literary expression which enables her to impress her original ideas on other people."[141] These positive attributes were moderated by the fact that "if the work is routine & she hasn't the power to plan & think, she gets careless & indifferent & of course the original qualities which she possesses imply 'temperament,' whatever that means–but which in her case means nothing small."[142] Ending on a more positive note, Ellicott concluded that "sometimes I have found it necessary to show her the other side of a question but have always found her ready to co-operate."[143] Her mixed assessment of La Motte's personality was reinforced by Mary Goodwillie, who described La Motte as "a strong, capable woman with … a very pronounced character" who was not "difficult to get along with."[144] The qualities that made La Motte a successful nurse and executive–her intelligence, organizational ability, forthrightness, and eloquence–also made her potentially difficult because she lacked the malleable and retiring nature fostered in so many women who had come into adulthood–like the letter writers and La Motte–during the late nineteenth century.

Undoubtedly, her candor and outspokenness made her an effective suffrage campaigner–something that was perceived as being at odds with her first responsibility to her tuberculosis work, as implied by Gertrude W. Peabody, who did some investigative work for the IDNA. She interviewed Dr. Hurd of the Johns Hopkins Hospital, who confirmed the assessment of La Motte as having "decided executive ability … [and] a strong personality & strong opinions," without which, Peabody grudgingly admitted, "she wouldn't be a leader."[145] Peabody was very wary of the "powerful personality" and "the quality I have heard of in J.H.H. graduates–men & women that the J.H. way is right & every other wrong."[146] She added an additional caution: La Motte "is a rabid suffragist as is Miss Lent who was so carried away by the cause that she had to be spoken to by the V. N. [Visiting Nurse] authorities, but since then has been subdued."[147]

This depressing statement, intended to be reassuring, fortunately was an overstatement by Peabody. Perhaps it convinced Codman, for in a letter from Crandall she applauds Codman's decision "to secure Miss La Motte."[148] However, Crandall wrote her letter a day after Peabody wrote to Codman to suggest they proceed carefully with interviewing La Motte, which means that Crandall was probably mistaken in her belief that a final decision had been made to recruit La Motte. A second letter from Goodwillie supports this view: written on September 12, 1911, it offers more advice on how to learn more about La Motte, such as contacting Theo Jacobs, the woman running the Federated Charities in Baltimore, to discover "how Miss La Motte works with other organizations" and to offer her opinion that "La Motte is more co-operative than Miss Lent," an interesting observation given that La Motte was often portrayed in the Baltimore press as more of a hardliner with regard to suffrage and tuberculosis nursing than Lent. Lent herself weighed in with what could hardly be an objective assessment of La Motte, who had been her colleague and officemate at 1123 Madison Avenue, the headquarters of the IVNA; they were, according to Ellicott, "devoted friends."[149] Unsurprisingly, Lent gave La Motte a very positive reference, highlighting as others did before her her excellent executive capacity and "shrewdness, judgment, and tact."[150] Her only reservation was that she did not know if La Motte would be willing to leave Baltimore and her position with the health department. Certainly, James Bosley, Commissioner of Health, communicated his "concern" at the prospect of losing La Motte, who he believed possessed more "'ability, tact, and enthusiastic devotion' than any other woman that has come under my observation during my public life."[151]

It turns out that La Motte was not willing to leave Baltimore, because her work was "in too unsettled a state for me to leave it. It has not yet reached its highest degree of efficiency, nor is it even able to stand alone."[152] She repeated her refusal in a subsequent letter in reply to a second request from Codman, who, encouraged by Crandall, asked La Motte to reconsider. La Motte's arguments about why she could not leave Baltimore were consistent with those laid out in her first letter and augmented by her assertion that "I'm the only woman that has ever had charge of a city department here in Baltimore, & … simply have got to stay."[153] La Motte's devotion to Baltimore was understandable: she had made history by being the first woman named to lead a city department and the tuberculosis epidemic was still in full swing. Presumably, her well-developed network of colleagues, friends, and fellow suffragists also kept her in the place she had called home for many of the past thirteen years.

Although La Motte could not very well discuss her continued commitment to suffrage campaigning in her refusal letters to

Codman, she was well integrated into the ongoing suffrage movement in Baltimore and would have been loath to leave an environment in which she had a voice and mechanisms for making herself heard. One of those was the *Maryland Suffrage News*, the publication started by Hooker to fill the void left by the *New Voter* a year earlier. It began publication on April 6, 1912, serving as an important resource for all suffrage-related activities and campaigning in the state. In the first issue, the editors explained the purpose of the journal: "its aims and purposes are to give the news of suffrage activity in this State, to afford Maryland Suffragists, irrespective of league affiliation, a medium in which they can discuss the phases and developments of the cause … and to help in shaping and directing the fight for the enfranchisement of the women of Maryland."[154] While the focus was on state activities, like the *New Voter*, it was keen to link itself to larger national and international suffrage issues and did so by stating on its masthead that it was a "supplement to *The Woman's Journal*," the national publication started by Lucy Stone and her husband Henry Blackwell in 1870 as a conservative response to the *Revolution*, the journal of the National Woman Suffrage Association.[155] La Motte assumed an official role with the paper with the December 28, 1912 issue, when she became a contributing editor,[156] but her name was in print in its pages before her official association–for example, she is listed as an available speaker for parlor meetings as early as the paper's second issue.[157]

One of the first significant events for which the paper was used to generate interest was Baltimore's first suffrage parade in June 1912. La Motte was at the heart of this event, having been named the chief marshal.[158] In the six weeks preceding the parade, originally scheduled for June 27, the paper gave frequent updates on the progress of its organization, listed committed participants, and asked for funds to support the many costs associated with the floats, banners, and renting of horses that formed an integral part of the parade. La Motte provoked debate when she published "The Wedding Guests," a reference to the parable of the great banquet in Matthew 22:1–14, and asserted that "to some of us who have the matter deeply at heart a parade seems a fitting opportunity for showing our colors, for testifying publicly to that which we believe, even if to do so means some sacrifice on our part."[159] In contrast, she wrote, "there are others, however, who will not join us–people on whom we had counted, whose ideals had always seemed so true and fine that it was impossible to doubt them–yet this parade business is showing up the value of these with startling directness."[160] Her direct condemnation of proclaimed suffragists who refused to participate must have been intended to bring forth public responses from the accused, a mechanism to encourage debate and draw attention to the parade.

If so, it had the desired effect: Elizabeth King Ellicott castigated La Motte in a letter to the editor in which she wrote that she "has seen fit to introduce a self-constituted test of true suffragists in regard to participation in the coming parade … injustice of the most pronounced type is evident in this article."[161] According to Ellicott, what would promote suffrage in the long run was "steady judgment [and] persistent effort" on the part of "Maryland suffragists who are quietly working for the solid strength of suffrage, but who cannot convince themselves that it is their duty to join a parade during a week of practical national issues, when, in addition to the greatest statesmen in the Democratic party, a horde of questionable characters are looking for every means to promote excitement."[162] Ellicott, whose devotion to the cause no one could question, uses rhetoric that smacks of a Victorian aversion to women raising their voices or mixing in public with potentially contaminating influences, highlighting the more conservative approach exercised by her and the Equal Suffrage League. Her view was reinforced by Lilian Welsh, who called La Motte's editorial "disappointing" and "distasteful" for the way it broke with ranks and criticized fellow suffragists in public.[163] For all of her dislike of La Motte's rhetoric, however, Welsh conceded that she had "made a mistake in judgment" in thinking the timing of the parade was "inopportune and the expense unjustifiable," because after watching it she found "that the parade served an important function in public education."[164] Welsh was so inspired by what she saw that she ended up marching in the Congressional Union parade in March 1913, an event surrounded by much more controversy than the Baltimore parade. "The Wedding Guests" resurfaced in a piece by Edith Houghton Hooker the next month in which she challenged Ellicott's reading, stating that the "test" of the suffragists was not whether they would participate in the parade, something she saw as "a matter of personal choice and convenience," but whether they would "pull together in an undertaking which involves the common cause, even at the cost of sacrificing one's dignity and better judgment."[165]

Hooker could afford to occupy a confrontational position post-parade. Most observers and commentators concurred with Welsh's assessment of its positive outcomes. It made an impression on journalists covering it–the parade was hailed as "the greatest suffrage parade in Maryland"[166]–and thousands of people marched and watched along the parade route. La Motte was at the literal heart of the parade at Mount Vernon Place, where she stood at the center of groups, lined up at the intersection on the square, representing different states. She, true to character, took her job seriously and expected those marching to do the same. Her "Directions for Marshals" communicated the gravity of their task, instructing them to make sure marchers walked "four abreast" in "banks six feet apart."[167] They were also "to keep eyes front … walk in a dignified manner; not to talk, laugh, chew gum, or speak to people along the route."[168] La Motte herself walked alongside Dr. Anna Howard Shaw, the president of NAWSA,[169] as a woman dressed as Joan of Arc and mounted on horseback led other women on horses, in chariots, and on foot to the convention hall where the 1912 Democratic National Convention was taking place.

The coverage in the *Maryland Suffrage News* was exuberant. Having overcome the disappointment of cancelling the parade on June 27, a move which angered some participants who had taken hours off of work to be there, they were relieved that the weather on the 28th allowed for marching and reported that it was "the best parade in Maryland."[170] La Motte gave her own report on its success, noting that "possibly no keener enjoyment of the entire parade was had than by" the grand marshal and her assistants, Dr. Florence Sabin and Mrs. Howard Schwartz: "certainly reviewing the parade for its entire length, and then walking ahead and letting it pass by again, was a delight … It was with difficulty that Mrs. Schwartz was restrained from bursting among the spectators and asking, 'Isn't it simply glorious?' FOR IT WAS."[171]

La Motte's activities, professional and political, slowed down later that summer when she had to have emergency surgery for appendicitis.[172] She was accompanied to the hospital by Lent, described as her "co-worker … and her almost constant attendant."[173] At this point, Lent and La Motte had a relationship stretching back as far as at least 1905, when La Motte joined the IVNA, and the two had served as sources of support for each other in times of illness and worked closely in the suffrage campaign as well. If their relationship exceeded that of close friends, the evidence is bare: in a November 1913 letter from La Motte, who was now living in Paris, to Wesselhoeft von Erdberg, she reflected "I think you are right about Mary. This separation has brought a better understanding and I find that my love for her all these years is very real."[174] This scant reference in all probability was to Lent, from whom La Motte had been separated for five months at this point and who received mail for her and helped her with her correspondence while she was overseas for several years. The two used 1123 Madison Avenue, the home of the IVNA, as their address for years and Lent may have been the person opening the letters La Motte received from "Louise" in the fall of 1911. She explained to Wesselhoeft von Erdberg that "every letter she wrote me was opened and copied, and I was being hounded to throw her over,– with the alternative offered."[175] These cryptic lines do not lend clarity to La Motte's trying situation other than to highlight that her relationship with "Louise" was perceived as a threat by someone probably motivated by jealousy.

Whatever the terms of their relationship, La Motte, once recovered from surgery, and Lent continued to campaign side by side with many other Maryland women to promote their belief in the importance and eventuality of suffrage. The successful parade of June 1912 immediately led to planning for a future parade to be held the next spring. Using the *Maryland Suffrage News* as her vehicle, La Motte returned to a topic about which she felt passionately: the injustice of the law. In "Fine Day," she describes 250 women being called into court to pay fines of $5 each for running brothels. La Motte bemoans the ludicrousness of fining them only to let them loose again to resume their business. The piece is full of rich detail as La Motte describes the assorted group of women: "some were fat and gross, and expensively dressed; some were thin, bent, shabby, with ludicrous, old-fashioned bonnets. Some of the women were young; mere girls of 19 or 20. Others were old, and seemed to totter as they walked."[176] Despite breaking the law and exploiting vulnerable women in their brothels, they were painted in a sympathetic light by La Motte, with much of her compassion emerging from her knowledge that the women were being treated hypocritically by the police and the court. Homing in on one particularly terrified woman, La Motte struck up a conversation with her, discovering that the woman swore she had not kept a brothel for six months but was powerless to protest the fine because she was subject to the absolute authority of the officer charging her and the judge who "takes his word."[177] La Motte angrily questions how it was possible for "the judge and State's Attorney" to rely on "any man in a blue uniform who chooses to inform against" a woman.[178] Worse, she contends, is that while the women are held responsible for running the brothels, supplying the demand for female flesh, those making the demand are not guilty. In a favorite rhetorical move, she ends with a probing question: "the honorable judge upon the bench, the machinery of our courts, the authority of our Police Department–these things which we are taught to respect–are they not all a party to this hypocrisy; to this travesty on honor and on justice?"[179] This attack brought a reply from the judge himself, who was "tempted to call [La Motte] before the Grand Jury and ask her to explain upon what basis she wrote that article."[180] The article quoted La Motte's piece at length and invited Judge Elliott to explain why he did not favor dismantling the bordello districts, a cause for which La Motte, Hooker, and others writing for the *Maryland Suffrage News* campaigned hard. Elliott makes familiar arguments about the importance of containing "the social evil" and complains that the women working in the brothels should be taught "they are leading immoral lives."[181] He remained typically silent on the part of the men creating demand for their services.

Never one to back down from conflict, no matter how public, La Motte was not cowed by this public castigation of her reporting techniques or her views of legalized prostitution. In a follow-up article, she proclaimed her readiness to appear before the Grand Jury and called Elliott's argument regarding the benefits of tolerating prostitution "idiotic."[182] Her solution was to "shut every disorderly house at once. If the keeper moves elsewhere, follow her and repeat the closing process."[183] If her recommendation resulted in the turning out of prostitutes onto the streets, she was fully in favor for "then the shame will be patent to all."[184] An additional benefit would be that exposing "the double standard whereby men feel free to do what they forbid their women will cure street-walking and with it prostitution."[185] La Motte's penchant for drastic action, something established with her position regarding the need to institutionalize tuberculosis patients,[186] and willingness to sacrifice individuals for the benefit of the many was also articulated in her answer to the interviewer's question regarding the danger of driving "women of lewd lives out into the home districts of the working classes."[187] She professed that "some must suffer always in this world that good may be attained," thereby distancing herself from the stereotypical sentimental reformers she found "disgusting" for naively believing that abolishing the brothel districts would lead to the end of prostitution.[188]

The focus of her writing for the *Maryland Suffrage News* in the fall and winter continued to be on the hypocrisy of Baltimore's handling of houses of prostitution, and she lashed out at the double standard of recording the intimate details of the women who work in such houses while acquiring no details about the men who visit them. She asked, "wouldn't it be a fair deal to send in to police headquarters such … information concerning every man who patronized the house–name, age, color of eyes and hair … The only objection we can urge against it would be that of economy–the expense of printing all those blanks."[189] She also published small follow-up pieces documenting the written laws of the city, how they were actually upheld and interpreted by the police with regard to prostitution, the way the courts continued to treat those arrested for maintaining brothels, and how the city benefited economically from the practices of fining those running "bawdy houses" but refused to move to shut them down permanently. In a surprising revelation, she documented how seven of the city's dispensaries received their funding through the fines levied against the brothel keepers once a year on "Fine Day," demonstrating that there was a network of complicity with the practice of tolerating the presence of these illegal establishments: ultimately the money collected would partially benefit the charities taking care of the sick and indigent of Baltimore, undoubtedly some of them having become sick because of their work in or visits to the very houses that would eventually contribute toward their care. Tracing the level of corruption further, La Motte revealed that the dispensaries were not the only beneficiaries of the fining system: the State's Attorney's Office, the Clerk of the Court, and the Sheriff's office also received more than $3,700 on Fine Day.[190] The hypocrisy of the system was too much to bear for La Motte, who commented, "there is such a locking and interlocking between honor and dishonor, truth and hypocrisy, justice and injustice, law-makers and breakers, that one gets bewildered and confused to a degree."[191] She persisted with this topic, despite the overwhelming interests supporting the existence of the brothel system, until the end of the year, when she published one of her last signed pieces on the topic in which she preempted the arguments against her position, sarcastically charging the "vice-crusaders" and the "reformers" for "dragging all this disgusting business into the limelight" and "uncovering spiritual sewers" that should be "out of sight."[192] Her tone drips with cynicism as she pretends to take the innocent's point of view on why tolerating the hypocrisy of permitting brothels in the segregated system was preferable to exposing profoundly unjust and unsavory practices, all in the name of protecting people from having to face the realities of the corrupt nature of policing and the courts.

After the New Year, La Motte wrote less, or anyway is identified as writing less, in the pages of the *Maryland Suffrage News*. Her last signed piece was titled "A Confession," and served as one of several *mea culpas* by women prominent in the suffrage campaign in Baltimore about why they were wrong to have supported partial suffrage. It is a brilliant example of La Motte's scathing tone, typically directed outward toward those she regarded as ridiculous or hypocritical, this time used to evaluate her past actions. She looks back at the attempts in the winter of 1911/1912 to gain the vote with two bills presented to the Maryland Legislature: "one was for State-wide, universal suffrage for women on the same terms that it is given to men; the other was a bill asking for limited suffrage–limited to the taxpaying women of Baltimore."[193] The inevitable result was "the suffrage forces were divided" and both bills failed. She explained her decision to back a bill for partial suffrage with which she did not intellectually agree as "a mistake, an error in judgment which we have never ceased to regret."[194] It was a betrayal to support an example of "class legislation," and "it becomes difficult to explain" when "one has done much talking about the value of the ballot if conferred on working women, women in the home, women in the courts, and so forth."[195] The explanation she gave at the time was that "it was rather lamely explained by saying tha[t] an enfranchised class would act as leaven on the community," and she "clung desperately to the idea of the entering wedge and our personal desire to vote before we became senile."[196] She then more fully owns up to her personal aspirations and desires–herein enters the confession–that "in spite of this excess of altruism, somewhere in the hinterland of consciousness lay the flicker of an idea. Property, a house, taxes; and then triumphal entry into the polling booth."[197] She imagined buying "a tumbledown, rat-ridden den," which she could rent "at the highest rate we could wring out of it … to an overdriven, underpaid wreck of the working classes, the sort of woman whom we had so freely talked about as needing the ballot to protect her labor and her home."[198] In the end, she has to admit that "we had not meant to be a hypocrite, but we had deceived ourselves,"[199] and thanked the very politicians who had undoubtedly enraged her when they refused to support the proposed suffrage bills.

La Motte's declaration that she was henceforth backing the more radical position of suffrage for all women, combined with her public conflict with a judge and her declaration that she was "not a reformer,"[200] indicates that she was feeling restless in her community and willing to take risks that might lead to ruptures with her network of fellow activists. Perhaps to channel some of that energy and desire for the new, she continued to participate in mass demonstrations of women's political will by volunteering to participate in a suffrage hike from Baltimore to Washington, DC with General Jones' army.[201] Though she and others, including Lent, Dixon, and Hooker, put their names on the list of hikers and are featured prominently on the cover of the *Maryland Suffrage News* dressed as hikers (see Figure 4), it is unlikely La Motte made the journey, because she was aiding Lent during her post-surgery convalescence; in addition, the enthusiasm of the hikers waned due to conflict between Jones and her group and the local suffragists. According to local coverage, which seemed to revel in potential discord between the groups and mocking the aspirations of the Baltimore hikers, Jones' group had refused the hospitality planned by the local suffrage organizations because "the hike is not a social affair."[202] Jones also is recorded as observing that "now that they [local suffragists] have learned how rough is the way and how fast our speed," she was not sure how long they would persist.[203] Whether La Motte walked to Washington is unclear, though she is credited with being the Grand Marshal of the Maryland division in coverage by the *Maryland Suffrage News*, though if she was, the publication is strangely silent on her involvement (see Figure 5).

SATURDAY, JANUARY 25, 1913

MARYLAND HIKERS

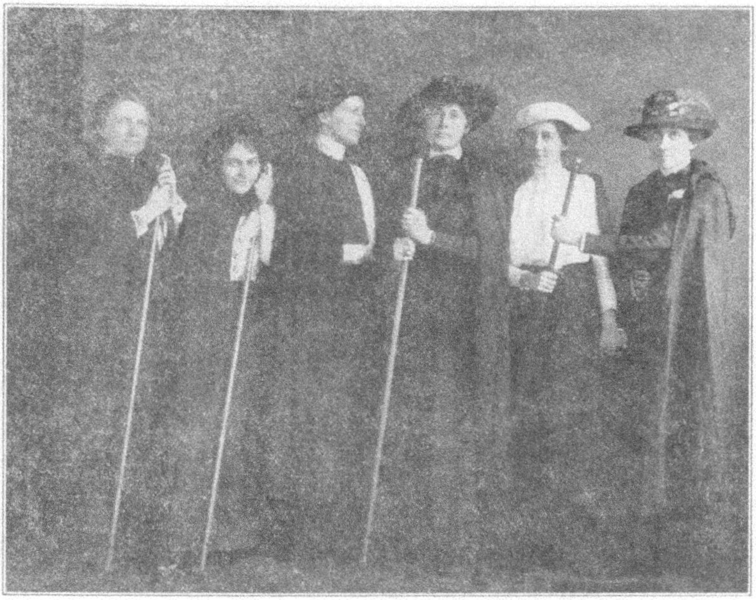

THOSE WHO HAVE ENLISTED IN GENERAL JONES' ARMY.

From left to right—Mrs. Frank Ramey, Mrs. C. J. Keller, Mrs. D. R. Hooker, Miss Ellen LaMotte, Miss M. B. Dixon, Miss M. E. Lent.

Figure 4 "Maryland Hikers," *Maryland Suffrage News*, January 25, 1913

La Motte eventually found broader vistas and more radical company when she opted to combine her political and writing interests by serving as a "special correspondent" to the *Sun* in a series of articles written to inform both sides of the debate about the activities of militant suffragettes in England.[204] In an interview, she discussed her reasons for taking "an indefinite furlough" from nursing: she was "stale" and needed a break from the routine of work.[205] Prodded by the interviewer about possibly embracing militant tactics herself, La Motte clarified that she intended "to go there and watch from the side lines" and to become more familiar with these women she much

SATURDAY, MARCH 15, 1913

GRAND MARSHAL OF MARYLAND DIVISION OF THE WASHINGTON PARADE-PAGEANT

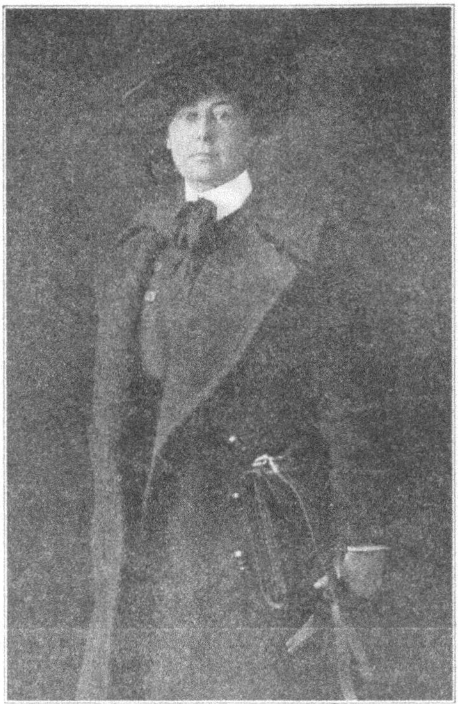

Holmes & Bishop.

Miss LaMotte is a graduate of the Johns Hopkins Training School for Nurses and is in charge of the Municipal Tuberculosis Work

Figure 5 La Motte, "Grand Marshal of Maryland Division of the Washington Parade-Pageant," *Maryland Suffrage News*, March 15, 1913

admired, for they "have shaken off the conventionalities which have bound [*sic*] them down for years."[206] While looking for a break from her work and for a change of scenery, La Motte was also clearly unsatisfied with the conservative approach to suffrage that was favored by her Baltimore colleagues. In 1913 Alice Paul and Lucy Burns, both of whom had worked with the Pankhursts in England, where they learned militant tactics, were revitalizing the activities of NAWSA via the Congressional Committee, including organizing the suffrage parade held the day before President Wilson's inauguration. La Motte was aware of their robust efforts as evidenced by her interest in participating in this parade, yet their activities were not enough to keep La Motte's attention. On June 20, 1913, she left Baltimore, sailing for England, where she spent the summer watching, but also participating in, a series of militant actions.

The articles La Motte wrote for the *Sun* document La Motte's attendance at numerous suffrage events and her move from observer to active participant as she got caught up in scuffles when police arrested prominent militant speakers. Her first report documents her disappointment after her arrival in London on June 30 at not finding any coverage of the militants' activities until she realized there was a "press boycott" on covering them. Her search for action took her to the recently raided offices of the WSPU, where she found things in tremendous disorder after the police had "smashed typewriters, upset filing cabinets and destroyed as much property as possible" while searching for "incriminating evidence against the suffrage leaders," which they had not found.[207] Having learned that Sylvia Pankhurst was to give a talk on July 3, she attended the meeting and heard Pankhurst describe her determination to maintain a hunger strike should she be arrested for "hoot[ing] the Cabinet," after a charge of "inciting to riot" had been brought against her.[208] La Motte attended her trial on July 5 and there met Mary Richardson. If La Motte was truly looking to make connections with the militant community, she could have done no better than establishing a relationship with Richardson, who was regularly involved in their activities and eventually became infamous for slashing the "Rokeby" *Venus* by Velázquez in the National Gallery in London in March 1914.[209] She became La Motte's guide to the suffragette community; the two of them escaped unscathed from a riot that occurred when Pankhurst, who never showed for her trial, tempted fate several days later and gave a talk in the East End of London. Despite leaving the building in groups of three with linked arms and singing a revised version of "La Marseillaise," a mêlée broke out as the police tried to disperse the group to find Pankhurst, who was successfully arrested that evening.

The reaction in Baltimore to her first missive was undoubtedly mixed: the *Maryland Suffrage News* was silent on the piece, while the *Sun* printed a scathing letter from Mrs. Josephine Grasett, a British woman who took La Motte to task, declaring any woman who "prefers to stand shoulder to shoulder with men in the world's daily struggles," an object of "contempt."[210] Grasett attacked La Motte's femininity, arguing that "a true woman respects a manly man and loves the master in him. She is proud of his protection, his power. I said a *true* woman–not the feather head beyond control, not the man-woman nor the boastful bachelor girl, but the tender, clinging vine, the motherly, capable girl helpmeet, chum companion, anyone who rejoices in motherhood and honors it before the 'cause,' who glories in her submission as wife to a real man."[211] While these arguments may have reverberated with the conservative members of Baltimore's community, the familiar attacks on the value and worth of any woman who dared to raise her voice in public cannot have bothered La Motte, who never strove to be a "clinging vine" and took great pride in her intellect and capacity for independent action. Mary Richardson rushed to La Motte's defense in a letter written on August 15 and published in the *Sun* on August 29. She unsurprisingly challenged why Grasett, proud of her family's military background, could not condone "the militant principle being employed by women, for if a theory stands right in principle it does not matter which sex employs it."[212] She also defended La Motte's sketch of the police as capable of violence and following the order "not to arrest, but terrify women," actions which demanded only one response: militancy.[213]

That interest in tracing the activities of women like herself who were determined to claim their political rights persisted during La Motte's months in England, when she became more familiar with the motivations of the women engaged in dangerous work for the movement. She had tea with several pseudonymously named women and interrogated them about why they would choose to put themselves at risk and violate the law instead of trying "other methods–sane argument, logical reasoning, the gradual winning over to your point of view."[214] Their response highlighted their fatigue with being "ladylike" after trying all legal methods for fifty years.[215] No longer asking for "the vote," they clarified that they were demanding "justice–simple justice and political equality" and were met with "curtailment of free speech, free press, the liberty of selling papers on the streets … [and] being arrested on trumped-up charges."[216] They were willing to endure cruelty, injustice, prison, and the loss of family and friends in order to create a more equal and just society and had lost faith that waiting patiently would bear fruit.

In a subsequent report, La Motte explained that the escalation of militancy came after "Black Friday," November 18, 1910, when women, bearing a petition and exercising their legal right to see the Prime Minister, were met with deliberate police brutality intended to terrorize and prevent them from continuing their efforts to deliver such petitions. The attempt to use force to cow women into abandoning the fight did not work but invigorated the militant effort, since suffragettes had "lost all respect for law, for authority, for a system under which human rights are treated with brutality."[217] La Motte herself was driven to give a man who was hitting an old woman in the face during the mêlée after Annie Kenney's arrest "a smash with a fist between the eyes."[218] She clearly reveled in the "intense exciting atmosphere" of meetings and activities of the WSPU and deliberately contrasted them with the "perfectly peaceful suffrage meetings" she was accustomed to, "where the sole emotion is apt to be boredom over the shopworn, if sound, arguments."[219] She testified in court against police brutality after being swept up in the riot, and saw injustice meted out when the judge, indifferent to the statement of those like herself who swore the police had treated the crowd with deliberate brutality, handed out the same sentence to the men and women accused by the police of assaulting them. For her, such a flagrant refusal to acknowledge the role of the police in terrorizing suffrage campaigners led to fomenting further militancy.

La Motte also wrote about more prosaic subjects, like selling copies of the *Suffragette*, after being charged to do so by Mary Richardson while she was serving her sentence in Holloway.[220] From her street-level perspective she had the chance to observe the depth of negative feeling many felt toward the suffragettes: "scorn, hatred, opposition of the most determined character."[221] La Motte received more than insults when several men stopped to deliver death threats to her, inducing her to ponder the root of the rage ignited by the movement in some men and women. She ends her article with a description of "a swaggering soldier, wearing the King's red uniform" who sends a "sneer" her way as he passes by, hitting her poster with "his little cane" because he "couldn't bear militancy."[222] This brief interaction leads La Motte to suggest that "militancy, when one wears his Majesty's uniform, and is paid for the taking of human life, is a different enterprise from militancy of a guerilla type, practiced by women, and having for its object the destruction of a system in which human life ranks low."[223] La Motte follows this acute observation with the following cogent question: "Can it be that destruction of property, for the preservation of human life, is a less noble thing than destruction of human life incident to the acquirement of property? So much depends on the viewpoint."[224] Her questioning of the meaning and purpose of militancy as it is engendered by male military service and (predominantly) female suffrage activities reveals the degree to which La Motte's understanding of the importance of suffrage was not limited to seeing the vote as a way to enact social housekeeping. In this piece she is not focused on the use of the vote but on the ideas about authority and power that perpetuate resistance to it.

La Motte continued to be involved with the militant suffrage movement after the summer of 1913, though in a more distant way. She hosted Mary Richardson in Paris for a week while she was recovering from her imprisonment. If Richardson had been a guide to militant suffrage activities for La Motte, La Motte took up her professional role as tuberculosis nurse to advocate on behalf of Richardson's health. In a letter to Christabel Pankhurst, La Motte describes her suspicion that Richardson is suffering from pulmonary tuberculosis made worse by the forced feedings to which she was subjected during several imprisonments at Holloway.[225] In this capacity La Motte is able to draw on her professional abilities to advocate for Richardson and by extension the suffrage cause. Her appeal received notice in *Votes for Women*, a British suffrage publication, only in it La Motte has become "Dr. Ellen La Motte, Mary Richardson's own medical attendant" and her letter is credited with launching an investigation into Richardson's health.[226]

While the actions of women like Richardson were heavily criticized by the British and Americans, La Motte perceived them as the logical outcome of being a member of a "fighting race."[227] In one of La Motte's final public statements on the subject, she returns to the examination of the connection between militancy and its incarnation in the actions of suffragettes. In her assessment, England's long history of warring and imperialism has logically resulted in women too possessing "courage, daring, and endurance."[228] That some women should choose to employ those characteristics in the service of the vote is a natural consequence of their heredity. This conceptualization of suffrage situates La Motte some distance from the position taken by Julia Rogers in 1910 regarding the "natural" timidity of southern women, and though La Motte was a southerner by birth, it is clear that her sympathies evolved to be with those women unafraid of raising their voices and even their fists if need be. Her ultimate assessment of militancy, however, was more qualified. Upon her return to Baltimore in August 1914, after fourteen months abroad, La Motte posited militancy a failure, not because of its methods but because it had lost force due to the intimidation of the government. With dwindling numbers, militants "can no longer intimidate, but, on the contrary, simply irritate the nation."[229] In addition, the impending war in Europe was shifting people's focus from the strife at home to conflict abroad, with the war ultimately re-ordering the priorities of both militants and "antis" alike. For La Motte, the war marked the end of her intense engagement with suffrage, initiated her career as a war nurse, and helped her to refine her analysis of militancy in the context of soldiering during the Great War.

Notes

1 Founded in 1903 by Emmeline Pankhurst, the WSPU employed militant tactics such as window smashing and arson in the effort to win the vote. For an overview, see E. Crawford, *The Women's Suffrage Movement: A Reference Guide 1866–1928* (London: UCL Press, 1999), pp. 727–755.

2 Ellen N. La Motte, "Ellen La Motte Insulted on Crowded London Street," *Sun* (September 28, 1913), p. M1.

3 See Chapter 1, n. 64, for more information about Lent.

4 "Praise for Judge Moses," *Sun* (January 7, 1910), p. 14.

5 "A Pretty Dance," *Scranton Republican* (January 21, 1893), p. 5.

6 "Wilmington Social Notes," *Times* (Philadelphia) (June 19, 1898), p. 7.

7 Sarah Hallenbeck, *Claiming the Bicycle: Women, Rhetoric, and Technology in Nineteenth-Century America* (Carbondale, IL: Southern Illinois University Press, 2016), p. 32.

8 "A Century Club Organized," *Evening Journal* (Wilmington, DE) (January 15, 1889), p. 3. For an extended discussion of the club, see Gail Stanislaw,

"Domestic Feminism in Wilmington: The New Century Club, 1889–1917," *Delaware History* 22:3 (1987), pp. 158–185.

9 Stanislaw, "Domestic Feminism," pp. 176–177.

10 Women from these families stand alongside her in the photograph, "Photograph of Women in Various National Costumes," 1898 (see Figure 2). In all likelihood, La Motte attended meetings of the club with them.

11 Anne Firor Scott, *Natural Allies: Women's Associations in American History* (Urbana, IL: University of Illinois Press, 1992), p. 142.

12 Social Service Club of Maryland (hereafter SSCMD), Maryland Historical Society, Baltimore, Maryland, *Minutes, 1906–1911.*

13 *Ibid.*

14 Dr. Claribel Cone (1864–1929) graduated from the Women's Medical College of Baltimore in 1890 and taught there as well. Ellen Hirschland and Nancy Hirschland Ramage, *The Cone Sisters of Baltimore: Collecting at Full Tilt* (Evanston, IL: Northwestern University Press, 2008) provides details about her life, work, and art collecting. Anna Herkner (est. 1879–1959) was a friend of La Motte's and appointed assistant to the chief of the Maryland Bureau of Industrial Statistics and Information in 1912. See Chapter 3 for a brief discussion of the controversy caused by her appointment and "Miss Herkner Dies: Fought Child Labor," *Sun* (December 4, 1959), p. 40+, for a biography. Dr. Lilian Welsh (1858–1938) graduated from the Women's Medical College of Pennsylvania in 1889 and joined the faculty of the Woman's College of Baltimore (Goucher College) in 1894. Her entry in the Maryland Women's Hall of Fame provides more information: https://msa.maryland.gov/msa/educ/exhibits/womenshall/html/welsh.html. Mary Bartlett Dixon Cullen (1873–1954) was a 1903 graduate of the Johns Hopkins Training Schools for Nurses and very involved in the suffrage movement. She later donated her suffrage materials to the Sophia Smith Collection, Smith College. Several letters in a private collection indicate Cullen and La Motte had contact as late as the 1950s; the two had been on friendly terms in the 1910s. Reba Thélin Foster, a 1903 graduate of Johns Hopkins, was the first nurse assigned to visit tuberculosis patients in Baltimore; see Ethel Johns and Blanche Pfefferkorn, *The Johns Hopkins Hospital School of Nursing 1889–1949* (Baltimore, MD: Johns Hopkins Press, 1954), p. 140, and served as the Just Government League's state organizer until 1913; see "Just Government League Organizer to Leave Baltimore," *Maryland Suffrage News* 2:26 (September 1913), p. 205. See Chapter 1, n. 64, for more information about Mary E. Lent.

15 Dr. Henry Hurd (1843–1927) was the first director of the Johns Hopkins Hospital and Dr. William Welch (1850–1934) was one of the founding professors of the Johns Hopkins Hospital. Julia Lathrop (1858–1932) was a social reformer and the first woman to head a federal bureau when she was appointed to the United States Children's Bureau in 1912.

16 SSCMD.
17 *Ibid.*
18 *Ibid.*
19 *Ibid.*
20 *Ibid.*
21 *Ibid.*
22 *Ibid.*
23 *Ibid.*
24 *Ibid.*
25 *Ibid.*
26 *Ibid.*
27 *Ibid.*
28 "Proceedings of the Eleventh Annual Convention of the Nurses' Associated Alumnæ of the United States," *AJN* 8:10 (July 1908), p. 860.
29 *Ibid.*
30 "Suffrage League Launched," *Sun* (January 29, 1909), p. 14.
31 "Mrs. Pankhurst's Address to Our Fair Suffragists," *Sun* (November 8, 1909), p. 4.
32 *Ibid.*
33 "Men in Suffrage Fight," *Sun* (January 4, 1910), p. 8.
34 *Ibid.*
35 Mary Bartlett Dixon Scrapbooks (hereafter MBDS), Suffrage Collection, Sophia Smith Collection, Smith College, Northampton, MA, "Will Not Support Radical Attitude," *Baltimore News*, undated.
36 "Mrs. Snowden Eloquent," *Sun* (November 28, 1909), p. 12.
37 "Women for the Ballot," *Sun* (December 6, 1909), p. 14. Presumably, this organization became the Just Government League, since all subsequent references to Lent's serving as president of a suffrage league are in relation to it.
38 "To Plan Suffrage Fight," *Sun* (January 7, 1910), p. 14.
39 "Nurses Become Suffragists," *Sun* (February 12, 1910), p. 7.
40 "'Give Us Votes!' the Cry," *Sun* (February 17, 1910), p. 9.
41 *Ibid.*
42 *Ibid.*
43 *Ibid.*
44 "Suffragists Sure They've Won the Vote," *Baltimore News* (February 17, 1910), p. 2.
45 Robert J. Brugger, *Maryland: A Middle Temperament, 1634–1980* (Baltimore, MD: Johns Hopkins University Press, 1988), p. 451.
46 MBDS, "Women Watchers Were on the Job," Scrapbook 1b, 1910.
47 MBDS, "Prospectus," *New Voter.*
48 "Eleventh Annual Report of the Alumnae Association of the Johns Hopkins Hospital Training School for Nurses, 1902–1903," *JHNAM* 2:3 (August 1903), p. 131.

49 MBDS, "Prospectus," *New Voter*.
50 I am using the term employed by the periodical, "suffragist."
51 Elizabeth King Ellicott, "Editorial," *New Voter* 1:1 (November 1910), p. 1.
52 "The Undercurrent of the Woman's Movement," *New Voter* 1:1 (November 1910), pp. 1–2.
53 Nurses in favor of suffrage often employed similar arguments. See S. B. Lewenson, *Taking Charge: Nursing, Suffrage and Feminism in America, 1873–1920* (New York: National Nursing League Press, 1996), especially pp. 138–178.
54 "The Undercurrent of the Woman's Movement," p. 2.
55 Nancy F. Cott discusses related issues in *The Grounding of Modern Feminism* (New Haven, CT: Yale University Press, 1987), p. 9.
56 "The Just Franchise League of Talbot Co, Maryland," *New Voter* 1:1 (November 1910), p. 4.
57 "Editorial. The Anti-Suffragists," *New Voter* 1:5 (January 1911), p. 37–38.
58 "The Conference for the Prevention of Infant Mortality," *New Voter* 1:2 (January 1911), p. 3.
59 *Ibid.*
60 "Editorial: (Women's) Suffrage for Men," *New Voter* 1:9 (April 1911), p. 72.
61 *Ibid.*
62 *Ibid.*, p. 73.
63 Mary Wollstonecraft, *A Vindication of the Rights of Men; A Vindication of the Rights of Woman; An Historical and Moral View of the French Revolution*, ed. Janet M. Todd (Oxford: Oxford University Press, 1999), p. 28.
64 *Ibid.*, p. 27.
65 See Marjorie Julian Spruill, "Race, Reform, and Reaction at the Turn of the Century: Southern Suffragists, the NAWSA, and the 'Southern Strategy' in Context," in J. Baker (ed.), *Votes for Women: The Struggle for Suffrage Revisited* (Oxford: Oxford University Press, 2002), pp. 102–117, for an overview of arguments regarding the role of race in southern women's campaigns for suffrage.
66 "A Central Legislative Committee," *New Voter* 1:5 (January 1911), p. 61.
67 "The Recognition of Woman," *New Voter* 1:8 (March 1911), pp. 61–62.
68 "Women's Suffrage and Women's Wages," *New Voter* 1:9 (April 1911), p. 73.
69 See Chapter 1 for a discussion of some of La Motte's racist attitudes in relation to nursing.
70 "Says Politics Sways Courts," *Sun* (October 28, 1910), p. 14.
71 "Court Proceedings," *New Voter* 1:2 (December 1910), p. 9. While no author is listed, the first issue of the *New Voter* advertised that La Motte would be writing such a column for the paper.
72 Ida Husted Harper, *The History of Woman Suffrage*, vol. 6 (New York: National American Woman Suffrage Association, 1922), p. 264.

73 Trax gave a talk on April 10, 1911, to the Board of Police Matrons, the same month the column was published, suggesting she was the content expert for the April 1911 column, which discusses the rape of minors and the punishment their attackers received.
74 "Court Proceedings," p. 9.
75 *Ibid.*
76 *Ibid.*
77 Ellen N. La Motte, *The Tuberculosis Nurse*, History of American Nursing (1915; repr., New York: Garland Press, 1985), pp. 117–118. Italics in the original.
78 "Court Proceedings," p. 10.
79 "Justice," *New Voter* 1:8 (March 1911), p. 65.
80 *Ibid.*
81 "Justice," *New Voter* 1:3 (December 1910), p. 27. Italics in the original.
82 "Justice," *New Voter* 1:9 (April 1911), p. 77.
83 *Ibid.*
84 *Ibid.*, p. 78.
85 *Ibid.*
86 "Justice," *New Voter* 1:10 (May 1911), p. 85.
87 *Ibid.*, p. 86.
88 *Ibid.*
89 "Justice," *New Voter* 1:3 (December 1910), p. 27.
90 *Ibid.*
91 "The Junior Suffrage League," *New Voter* 1:4 (January 1911), p. 32.
92 MBDS, "Letter from Board of Directors to Members of the Equal Suffrage League." If the organization put out these bulletins, none have been found.
93 "News Notes," *JHNAM* 10:3 (September 1911), p. 116.
94 "Louise" is mentioned in La Motte's letters to Amy Wesselhoeft von Erdberg, of which there are sixteen in the JHMI, Ellen N. La Motte Collection.
95 In her 1958 will, La Motte left Rosett $15,000, but in a 1961 codicil, she changed the amount to $5,000. See Probate Court, District of Columbia, "Last Will and Testament of Ellen N. La Motte."
96 The school is still in operation; see www.gilman.edu/about/history/archives for more information about its history.
97 "Dinner Before the German," *Sun* (December 5, 1905), p. 14.
98 "Personal," *Sun* (October 17, 1908), p. 6.
99 "Society Girls on Stump," *Sun* (May 28, 1910), p. 7.
100 "The Junior Suffrage League."
101 Edith Houghton Hooker was a prominent suffragist and social hygienist who trained as physician at John Hopkins. For more information about her, see the biographical note in the Maryland State Archives: http://msa.maryland.gov/megafile/msa/speccol/sc3500/sc3520/013600/013609/html/13609bio.html.
102 "Planks for the Cause," *Sun* (January 22, 1911), p. 8.

103 *Ibid.*
104 *Ibid.*
105 JHMI, "Ellen N. La Motte to Amy Wesselhoeft von Erdberg," December 19, 1911.
106 "Miss Carey Chooses Work," *Sun* (June 8, 1911), p. 16.
107 "Miss Carey Resigns," *Sun* (October 3, 1911), p. 8.
108 JHMI, "Ellen N. La Motte to Amy Wesselhoeft von Erdberg," December 19, 1911.
109 *Ibid.*
110 *Ibid.*
111 *Ibid.*
112 *Ibid.*
113 *Ibid.*
114 JHMI, "Ellen N. La Motte to Amy Wesselhoeft von Erdberg," December 23, 1911.
115 *Ibid.*
116 *Ibid.*
117 *Ibid.*
118 *Ibid.*
119 *Ibid.*
120 *Ibid.*
121 JHMI, "Ellen N. La Motte to Amy Wesselhoeft von Erdberg," March 20, 1912.
122 "'Baltimore Brieux' Talks of Socialism and Other Things," *Sun* (August 31, 1913), p. 17.
123 "Rosett's First Wife Assents," *Sun* (December 23, 1913), p. 7.
124 "Fashionable Philanthopy's Love Trail," *Pittsburgh Press* (January 18, 1914). This florid account gives the flavor of the press coverage of their engagement. On the same day that story was published, the *Sun* published a short piece announcing that the wedding had been postponed because Carey had had "a nervous breakdown." The article also reported that Rosett was twice her age when in fact he was about thirteen years her senior, making the factual content of these reports difficult to assess. See "Socialist's Romance Halted," *Sun* (January 18, 1914), p. 10. The two married in February, an event fraught with drama that the *Sun* covered in great detail. See "Miss Carey Weds Dr Joshua Rosett," *Sun* (February 8, 1914), p. 1+. Interest was revived in 1936 when the couple filed for a divorce in Reno, NV. See "Exciting Romance of 1914 Will End in Reno Divorce," *Sun* (November 18, 1936), p. 24+.
125 See Chapter 1 for a discussion of La Motte's professional activities after being hired by the Baltimore Health Department.
126 JHMI, "Ellen N. La Motte to Amy Wesselhoeft von Erdberg," March 20, 1912.
127 *Ibid.*
128 MBDS, Elizabeth King Ellicott, "Reasons for Presenting Municipal Bills for the Enfranchisement of Taxpaying Women to the Maryland Legislature," 1912.

129 *Ibid.*
130 *Ibid.*
131 JHMI, "Ellen N. La Motte to Amy Wesselhoeft von Erdberg," March 20, 1912.
132 "'Tis Suffragists' Great Day," *Sun* (February 13, 1912), p. 12.
133 "Suffrage Bill Dead," *Sun* (March 1, 1912), p. 11.
134 *Ibid.*
135 *Ibid.*
136 "Politics and Nurses," *Sun* (February 21, 1910), p. 4.
137 *Ibid.*
138 *Ibid.*
139 "Here Are Words of Cheer and Praise," *Sun* (February 25, 1910), p. 4.
140 Instructive District Nursing Association of Boston Collection, Howard Gotlieb Archival Research Center, Boston University (hereafter IDNA), "Ella Phillips Crandall to Katharine B. Codman," August 31, 1911. Buhler-Wilkerson discusses the IDNA's attempts to hire La Motte. See Karen Buhler-Wilkerson, *False Dawn: The Rise and Decline of Public Health Nursing, 1900–1930* (New York: Garland, 1989), p. 55, n. 42, and pp. 59–60.
141 IDNA, "Elizabeth King Ellicott to Katharine B. Codman," undated.
142 *Ibid.*
143 *Ibid.*
144 IDNA, "Mary Goodwillie to Katharine B. Codman," September 13, 1911. Goodwillie (1873–1949) was involved in many civic improvement efforts in Baltimore and is in the Maryland Women's Hall of Fame: https://msa.maryland.gov/msa/educ/exhibits/womenshall/html/goodwillie.html.
145 IDNA, "Gertrude W. Peabody to Katharine B. Codman," September 8, 1911.
146 *Ibid.* This charge would certainly be brought against La Motte by Mortimer during World War One. See Chapter 4 for a discussion of their relationship.
147 *Ibid.*
148 IDNA, "Crandall to Codman," September 9, 1911.
149 IDNA, "Ellicott to Codman," undated.
150 IDNA, "Mary E. Lent to Katharine B. Codman," September 14, 1911.
151 IDNA, "James Bosley to Katharine B. Codman," September 21, 1911.
152 IDNA, "Ellen N. La Motte to Katharine B. Codman," September 23, 1911.
153 IDNA, "Ellen N. La Motte to Katharine B. Codman," October 3, 1911.
154 "In Which We Introduce Our Selves," *Maryland Suffrage News* 1:1 (April 1912), p. 2.
155 Martha Watson, *A Voice of Their Own: The Woman Suffrage Press, 1840–1910* (Tuscaloosa, AL: University of Tuscaloosa Press, 1991), p. 88.
156 See the list of editors in the *Maryland Suffrage News* 1:39 (December 1912), p. 154.
157 "Parlor Meeting Best Method of Reaching People," *Maryland Suffrage News* 1:2 (April 1912), p. 5.
158 "Information for Marchers," *Maryland Suffrage News* 1:12 (June 1912), p. 45.

159 "The Wedding Guests," *Maryland Suffrage News* 1:11 (June 1912), p. 42.
160 *Ibid.*
161 Elizabeth Ling Ellicott, "The Letter Box," *Maryland Suffrage News* 1:13 (June 1912), p. 50.
162 *Ibid.*
163 Lilian Welsh, "The Letter Box," *Maryland Suffrage News* 1:15 (July 1912), p. 58. Welsh (1858–1938) was a pioneering female physician and professor at Goucher College who was strongly committed to female suffrage.
164 *Ibid.*
165 "The Wedding Guests–Continued," *Maryland Suffrage News* 1:15 (July 1912), p. 70.
166 "March Like Men," *Sun* (June 29, 1912), p. 20.
167 MBDS, "Directions for Marshals," Scrapbook 4a, 1912.
168 *Ibid.*
169 "March Like Men," p. 20.
170 "The Baltimore Parade," *Maryland Suffrage News* 1:14 (July 1912), p. 55.
171 "Our Suffrage Parade as Seen by the Grand Marshal," *Maryland Suffrage News* 1:15 (July 1912), p. 60.
172 "Miss La Motte Under Knife," *Sun* (July 21, 1912), p. 12.
173 *Ibid.*
174 JHMI, "Ellen N. La Motte to Amy Wesselhoeft von Erdberg," November 22, 1913.
175 JHMI, "Ellen N. La Motte to Amy Wesselhoeft von Erdberg," December 19, 1911.
176 "Fine Day," *Maryland Suffrage News* 1:33 (November 1912), p. 132.
177 *Ibid.*
178 *Ibid.*
179 *Ibid.*
180 MBDS, "Judge Raps Critics of the Bench," December 5, 1912.
181 *Ibid.*
182 MBDS, "Willing to Back Charge," undated.
183 *Ibid.*
184 *Ibid.*
185 *Ibid.*
186 See Chapter 1 for a discussion of her controversial views on tuberculosis.
187 "Willing to Back Charge."
188 *Ibid.*
189 Ellen N. La Motte, "Nobody's Business," *Maryland Suffrage News* 1:35 (November 1912), p. 139.
190 *Ibid.*
191 Ellen N. La Motte, "Five Dollars and Costs," *Maryland Suffrage News* 1:38 (December 1912), p. 152.

192 Ellen N. La Motte, "Reasonable Objections," *Maryland Suffrage News* 1:39 (December 1912), p. 156.
193 Ellen N. La Motte, "A Confession," *Maryland Suffrage News* 1:52 (March 1913), p. 208.
194 *Ibid.*
195 *Ibid.*
196 *Ibid.*
197 *Ibid.*
198 *Ibid.*
199 *Ibid.*
200 "Willing to Back Charge."
201 "Baltimoreans to March," *Sun* (January 21, 1913), p. 5.
202 MBDS, "On to Capital Now," *Sun* (26 February 1913), p. 3.
203 *Ibid.*
204 "Ellen La Motte on London's Suffragette Problems," *Sun* (July 20, 1913), p. SOS1.
205 "Miss La Motte Plans to Nurse Militancy," *Sun* (June 15, 1913), p. SO8.
206 *Ibid.*
207 Ellen N. La Motte, "While Britain Prays, Her Militants Sing Their Hymns of War," *Sun* (July 27, 1913), p. LS1.
208 *Ibid.*
209 Rowena Fowler, "Why Did Suffragettes Attack Works of Art?," *Journal of Women's History* 2:3 (Winter 1991), p. 110. For more about Richardson, see H. Kean, "Some Problems of Constructing and Reconstructing a Suffragette's Life: Mary Richardson, Suffragette, Socialist and Fascist," *Women's History Review* 7:4 (December 2006), pp. 475–493.
210 Josephine Grasett, "Attacks Ellen La Motte on Her London Letter," *Sun* (August 3, 1913), p. LS1.
211 While this letter reads almost as satire now, Grasett represented a part of the population that felt compelled to protect traditional conceptions of masculinity and femininity against what they saw as a dangerous assault by deviant women and men. See S. Goodier, *No Votes for Women: The New York State Anti-Suffrage Movement* (Urbana, IL: University of Illinois Press, 2012) for an exploration of why women took a position against the vote for women.
212 Mary Richardson, "Letters to the Editor," *Sun* (August 29, 1913), p. 6.
213 *Ibid.*
214 Ellen N. La Motte, "Miss La Motte Takes Tea with Militant Leaders in London Town," *Sun* (August 10, 1913), p. 17.
215 *Ibid.*
216 *Ibid.*
217 Ellen N. La Motte, "Wherein Miss La Motte Forces Man to Assume Silly Position," *Sun* (August 31, 1913), p. B5.
218 *Ibid.*

219 Ellen N. La Motte, "Caught in Suffragette Riot, Ellen N. La Motte, of Baltimore, Is Knocked Down and Then–Well, She Writes about It," *Sun* (September 7, 1913), p. MA3.
220 La Motte, "Ellen La Motte Insulted," p. M1.
221 *Ibid.*
222 *Ibid.*
223 *Ibid.*
224 *Ibid.*
225 Henry Devenish Harben, Manuscripts Department, the British Library, London, "Ellen N. La Motte to Christabel Pankhurst," October 19, 1913.
226 "Released after a Fortnight's Torture," *Votes for Women* 7:295 (October 1913), p. 67.
227 Ellen N. La Motte, "Miss La Motte Sees Reason in Blood," *Sun* (October 26, 1913), p. C16.
228 *Ibid.*
229 "No Faith in Militancy," *Sun* (August 12, 1914), p. 3.

3

In search of meaningful work, 1914–1915

An article published in Baltimore's the *Sun* in August 1914 recounts La Motte's thrilling return to the United States after an absence of seventeen months: she traveled on the *Minnetonka*, an Atlantic Transport liner, which, fearing an imminent attack by a German warship, had to take evasive maneuvers as it "ran for safety."[1] The liner docked without incident in New York City on August 10 and La Motte made her way to Baltimore, where she returned to the IVNA at 1123 Madison Avenue. Though she had resigned her position with the Baltimore Health Department in July 1914,[2] she undoubtedly returned to catch up with old friends and to decide in which direction she wanted to develop her professional life now that she had separated herself from her long-standing connections to nursing in Baltimore. Ultimately, whatever La Motte's plans may have been for her life after her return to the United States, the war shaped her decision to return as quickly as possible to France and to take up nursing to serve the country that had been her home for almost a year.

The Paris to which La Motte returned in October 1914 was much changed from what it had been when she set up her residence there in September 1913.[3] La Motte too had undergone a transformation in her focus and interests. Having completed her last report on militant suffragettes in London for the *Sun*, La Motte moved to Paris, where she determined to write her first book, published in 1915, the culmination of her professional nursing work, *The Tuberculosis Nurse*. This well-known subject matter, tuberculosis prevention and care, preoccupied her from September 1913 until early summer 1914.[4] While she was dealing with a very familiar topic during its composition, the location in which she was writing was dramatically different from the familiar streets of Baltimore. In Paris, she was exposed to a diverse world of artists who were experimenting with every possible art form and style. Living at 166, boulevard Montparnasse, La Motte was well situated in the Montparnasse district and familiar with the artists inhabiting the *quartier*. She felt ambivalent about being amongst this crowd and lamented in one letter that her friends were "a little too many for me .... They take up more of my time, and energy and nervous forces that I want to give. From being a perfectly lonely soul, I am swamped with invitations, which I can not resist nor refuse."[5] Her desire to isolate herself in order to make time to write drove her to leave Montparnasse and to take a room on the Île Saint-Louis where she imagined living in productive seclusion until the realities of living in a cold, smoke-filled room and being fed horse meat by her stingy *concierge* drove her back to her *pension* in Montparnasse within two weeks. As she explained to a friend, "I find my ability to work is dependent upon my being well. And sleep, food and fresh air are essentials."[6] While she liked to think she was cut out for living outside of the expensive and Americanized Montparnasse neighborhood, she had to admit that "Four generations have intervened between me and my ancestres [*sic*]–moreover, I believe they were people who were waited on to some extent, judging from my inherent inability to light a fire."[7] The comforts of familiar and warm surroundings were too much and she retreated to them no matter her persistent feeling that she needed to get away from the *quartier* and its "contaminating influences."[8]

La Motte's ambivalence toward her Parisian environment led her to be bemused, dismissive, and admiring of the eclectic crowd that habituated the cafés of the Left Bank. In one unfinished and unpublished story set in a café "on the border line of the Quartier Latin," the third-person narrator observes and assesses those around her, noting that it was "a motley crowd" of those "seeking ~~in this~~ retreat and sanctuary in this obscure café; others, and the majority, fancying themselves already famous, and emphasing [*sic*] strongly their eccentricities, real or cultivated; and still others, seeking in their ecentricities [*sic*] of dress and manner the last outward stand of a self assurance [*sic*] and self belief [*sic*] that had long since vanished. Pitiful shells they were."[9] This diversity and unconventionality undoubtedly engaged and sometimes repelled La Motte as it did so many others like her during the carefree years in Paris before the war, when Montparnasse was a magnet for artists, aspiring and established.

The apartment of American writer Gertrude Stein and her partner, Alice B. Toklas, was a hub for artistic and expatriate activity and conversation,[10] and Stein provided a gateway into avant-garde Paris, "introducing a lot of interesting people" to La Motte in the fall of 1913.[11] It is probable that La Motte and Stein met when Stein was studying at Johns Hopkins School of Medicine from the fall of 1897 until she left in 1902 without finishing her degree.[12] La Motte's diary also testifies that from January through March of 1915, when Stein and Toklas left for Spain, she visited them a half-dozen times. Most of the entries pertaining to Stein and Toklas say very little about the specifics of her observations of the couple other than to note that she found them "very entertaining"[13] and enjoyed a "charming lunch" with them on another occasion.[14] While she observes in a letter to Wesselhoeft von Erdberg that Stein "has a great collection of futurist pictures,"[15] she makes no specific comments about her reactions to being exposed to the art Stein collected.

Nonetheless, being exposed to avant-garde art, meeting artists and writers at Stein's, and reading Stein's own work had an influence on La Motte's reflections of narrative and writing.[16] Yet, during this period, she was in the midst of composing *The Tuberculosis Nurse*, a traditional textbook that would hardly have benefited from modernist innovation. La Motte saw her work on the book as "a duty" and was "terribly depressed" about finishing a draft of it because "it seems so inadequate and worthless and badly written and expressed–if that is the climax of all my years of work, what a commentary on them and me. I have done it so grudgingly, and it has been such mechanical uphill work."[17] The following month, after sharing her draft with friends, including the Clapps,[18] La Motte felt more hopeful, that "the book is not so bad as I at first thought … so that I feel somewhat encouraged."[19] That optimism would see her through the revision process and publication of the book in 1915; she eventually assessed the book after seeing it in published form as "a nice book," but "it is not really me,"[20] returning to the idea that she had written in out of a sense of obligation rather than passion.

Meanwhile, unpublished manuscripts reveal that she was also experimenting with multiple forays into fiction writing during this same period, a departure from her previous focus on writing about professional concerns related to nursing and social reform. In La Motte's *Drafts of Unfinished Stories and Sketches, 1911–1919*, there are a number of pieces she worked on from 1913 to 1914, some of which are meant to be amusing and light pieces, such as "The Coercion of Patricia," in which the first-person narrator uses her superior linguistic abilities in Italy to force her traveling companion, Patricia, to agree to get a cat when they return to Baltimore. A note by La Motte records that she sent the story to "M.E.L.," Mary E. Lent, La Motte's housemate, friend, and fellow nurse in Baltimore, when she completed it on June 24, 1914.[21] Lent acted as La Motte's go-between, forwarding mail for her and sending off manuscripts and contracts. It is possible La Motte intended for Lent to forward it to a magazine for review or she may have sent it to her as a gift. The two women had traveled together in Europe and lived and worked together for years. Given La Motte's penchant for drawing on her life experiences as the basis of her fiction, it is probable that the story incorporates some of her travels with Lent.

The story "Flea Fair" surely uses some of her personal explorations of Paris, specifically the *marché aux puces* at the Porte de Clignancourt. It draws strongly on La Motte's eye for detail as it describes the narrator's attempt to interest a group of well-to-do American women in accompanying her on a trip to the market. While they claim their hesitations stem from their fear of the filth and fleas they might encounter there, the narrator says, "Paris does one [of] two things to you–you either become inflexibly American and unyielding in your point of view, and preserve it against all the influences round about–or else you yield to the surrounding spirit of the French–and enjoy yourself."[22] Clearly, the narrator is a member of the latter group, as she sets off with an unnamed companion to investigate the fair and later marvels at "the earnestness of the peddlers, and the seriousness with which they offered things that could only have one use–to make a fire with."[23]

In another group of stories set in pre-war Paris, La Motte uses the city as a backdrop for characters searching for love or a way to infuse their lives with a sense of adventure or significance. In the improbably titled "Petria Smolianinoff," the first-person narrator, a writer whose gender is never identified, searches "the shifting crowds" of "the city … for my own."[24] The story traces the growing desire of the narrator to meet Smolianinoff after her name is uttered by a shared acquaintance. Yet, the narrator enjoys prolonging the moment of their meeting and anticipating the pleasure of the encounter with her, a sculptor living on the Left Bank who shares the narrator's certainty that they are destined for each other. The story is rare in La Motte's writings because of its exploration of sexual and romantic longing, yet it shares with other stories from the same period the use of the bohemian setting of the Left Bank to explore the mournful desires of other characters, such as American expatriates in "Les Transatlantiques." In this piece, the setting offers La Motte the opportunity, via the observant eye of the third-person narrator, to describe pre-war bohemian café culture, which she does by detailing the patrons of the café and their sometimes "shabby dress" and other times "bizarre, rather charming, artistic clothes" before focusing on a well-to-do American woman, sitting unaccompanied but evidently a frequent customer based on her friendly interactions with the waiter.[25] She draws the attention of an American man, also alone in the café, who is attracted to her, suspecting that she, like him, "knew the awful, grinding, homesick longing of one who has renounced his birthplace."[26] It is tempting to read into their conversation about their reasons for having left home some of La Motte's, particularly when the woman comments, "And when the judgement of those Others over There ran counter to mine, and would have compelled me into grooves that seemed to me cramped and false–then I could not live with them any more."[27] A letter to a friend written when La Motte was still working in Baltimore articulated her own willingness to cut all ties, personal and professional, for the woman she loved, "Louise":[28] "I told her that I would gladly give up my work here–without a question–all my friends, and every thing that I have gathered about myself … to go abroad."[29] Though "Louise" refuses La Motte, despite loving her, because of "social position and family pride," La Motte feels "singularly free" because she has "done [her] best to live up to whatever principles I believe in" and "my soul is free and honest."[30] "Les Transatlantiques" offers no resolution to the feelings of alienation and the longing for a place where the characters can realize their ideals; however, the story reflects La Motte's interest in using Paris as a backdrop for the exploration of desires both physical and emotional and provides a fictional venue for thinking through her wish to live a life in which she could fiercely adhere to her beliefs and feelings.

She takes on similar themes in "By-Products," while also weaving London, another city La Motte knew well, into the narrative. In this story, Sophie Cameron, an English sculptor living in Paris, is granted a small allowance by a rich but frugal uncle in London, Sir William Cameron, who has left Sophie to her own devices as she struggles to make a living in France. Sir William has only a few rules, one of which includes the requirement that if she marries, she must marry a man who can support her or he will stop sending her the allowance. Following a familiar melodramatic narrative, Sophie falls in love with a fellow struggling artist, the tenor Maurice Page, who makes the decision to leave her since he cannot support her with his art. He refuses Sir William's offer to employ him as a clerk in his brewing company, preferring to end his relationship rather than live a life of penury and sordidness, which, he believes, would result in the great love between him and Sophie deteriorating from a "great ideal" into "incessant struggle" and "petty details."[31] This story and "Les Transatlantiques" focus on the possibility of adhering to one's ideals, particularly ideals about the value of living unconventionally and loving without allowing economic realities to debase relationships. These stories, undoubtedly influenced by the unconventionality by which La Motte was surrounded in Montparnasse and her own search to live honestly, are preoccupied with personal quests for freedom and the place of the artist in society. While many other artists of the same period would explore these topics more effectively than La Motte in these unfinished drafts, she later returned to some of the exploration of the tenability of safeguarding one's ideals within the context of her writings about the Great War. In "By-Products," at one point Maurice Page gazes at the back gardens of the houses of the poor as his train approaches London: "He could not maintain his place in the flowing strem [*sic*] of civilization–he too belonged to that mass of waste material that gathers like froth on the edges of the rushing stream, the side wash of society."[32] The imagery of water, froth, and waste would be used more powerfully a few years later by La Motte in her incisive exploration of the meaning of modern war in *The Backwash of War*.

Despite the effort La Motte was putting forth during the winter of 1913/1914 to develop her skills as a creative writer, she either did not try or could not find a way to get her writings into print. Rather, the familiar territory of tuberculosis nursing would bear more fruit with the eventual publication of *The Tuberculosis Nurse*. Although La Motte may have intended to continue her writing efforts upon her return to the United States in the summer of 1914, the outbreak of the war drove her back to France in October 1914, and her desire to play a part in it kept her in Paris despite the many obstacles she had to overcome to find, after months of searching, a nursing position in a frontline hospital. That search is documented in the only surviving diary, covering much of 1915, kept by La Motte in 1915–1916. It is impossible to know if she kept other diaries and later destroyed them or they were lost, or if she decided to buy the T. J. & J. Smith's Foolscap Quarto Diary to commemorate her search for a frontline nursing position during this momentous time. Given her penchant for producing sketches of her patients, recording juridical proceedings in Baltimore, and doing various kinds of reporting, La Motte probably kept diaries or notebooks to help her flesh out her thoughts in the more formal kinds of writing she did. If so, these items are gone. The 1915 diary demonstrates that La Motte used it as a place where she could record her meetings with a wide assortment of expatriates and her dogged efforts to use her nursing skills to help the wounded. She rarely used it as an opportunity for self-exploration or self-reflection. While she only occasionally voiced her own intimate feelings, she did record her impressions of others, often giving way to her exasperation, derision, and sometimes pleasure as she had encounters with artists, socialites, and later nurses and others working in a hospital near the front lines in Belgium.

Early entries in the diary call attention to her frustration and sense of helplessness and uselessness during these months of running down opportunities to serve, only to be disappointed time and again. After a visit to Stein and Toklas, La Motte wrote in her diary:

> Feel very lost and desolate some how. It is all a failure, this effort of mine to be of use to France. Miss Toklas says that in the beginning there were scores of bluff, hearty Americans saying "Here is my …! My sympathies are with you–let me help". And they were so bluff, so hearty, so insistent that they became a nuisance. I suppose it is that way. We have "butted in" with our

> help, our service, long before we were asked or needed, & the French resent us. They want our money, but our service & interference, never! This point of view is very simple. The wounded get along as well without as with care, & better lose a legion without care, than risk a spy. After all, a wounded man is useless. He may as well be dead.[33]

La Motte's lamentation regarding her inability to find meaningful war work would be repeated in her diary over the next five months. During this period, La Motte bemoaned the fact that her nationality rendered her useless and that the French military had no understanding of the value of an expertly trained nurse. This indifference to and ignorance of her skills and even suspicion of her motives made her search to make a valuable contribution to the war a challenge professionally and personally.

An additional struggle for La Motte must have been her understanding of her professional nursing identity. After building a career from 1905 to 1913 in Baltimore and earning a reputation as an expert in the field of tuberculosis nursing,[34] La Motte left the security she had established for herself to start a new chapter in her life. She did have some financial support from her cousin, Alfred I. du Pont, but she had to manage on her own with a modest income, as evidenced by her moving in January 1915 to "a forlorn & shabbily furnished studio at 115, rue Notre-Dame-des-Champs."[35] Not only had she given up a regular income, she had also chosen to leave the sense of security and stability of living in a region where she was well established, with a strong network of colleagues, friends, and family, to inhabit a foreign country where she often felt unwanted and resented. Her desire to leave the career that had granted her independence and helped her to develop her professional voice as a writer and activist must have been strong indeed. Yet, with the start of the war, La Motte wanted to be of service and one of the few ways women could make an immediate contribution was through frontline nursing or ambulance driving. Given La Motte's extensive training as a nurse, her path was obvious though it did mean returning to the profession she had decided to quit, albeit in very different circumstances. Being a nurse once again had to become the identity she assumed as the way to find a place in the war.

La Motte and others undoubtedly realized that her skills and background could be put to good use by engaging in nursing once again, and while still in the USA in the late summer/early fall of 1914 La Motte was already making inquiries into opportunities to nurse in Europe and received an entreaty from one friend, Gertrude Austin, in Paris: "Come–American Ambulance."[36] The letter that followed Austin's cable explained that "the Head of the Nursing Staff, Miss Deveraux, has asked me to beg you to come and help us," but she warned that La Motte would have to prepare to find the work "very hard," something at which La Motte would later scoff.[37] While the *JHNAM* describes La Motte as taking charge of "the American Ambulance Service in connection with the Pasteur Hospital,"[38] La Motte says more modestly that she was "placed in charge of a small ward on the third floor, which had just been furnished and opened to receive patients."[39] The American Ambulance was a French military hospital "supported by American capital" and was a favorite destination for American volunteers because, in La Motte's caustic view, it was a place "where laymen and professionals, blundering or efficient, can work off their sympathies, their desire to help, or their desire to 'see things', with no questions asked as to impelling motives."[40] La Motte experienced other surprises at the American Ambulance when she realized that she would be working in "a modern hospital as large and almost as well equipped as the Johns Hopkins" and that she would be "on comfortable ten-hour duty, with two hours off a day, and a half day once a week, in a steam-heated, electric-lighted building with excellent food and a handful of patients."[41]

La Motte had prepared for "the hardships of war, the sufferings, the discomforts, the privation"[42] but was unsettled to find herself in a well-equipped hospital with more beds than patients. An additional source of astonishment was the presence of "auxiliaries … society women of the American colony in Paris," some of whom "are animated by a genuine desire to be of service, others by nothing more lofty than a craving for new sensations."[43] This excess of "unskilled labor," some of which La Motte deemed "useful, much superfluous, and some a positive menace to the patients," stood in stark contrast to the dearth of nurses, supplies, and beds available at the front.[44] At this point, La Motte had heard of the conditions near the front lines from English nurses who came to the Ambulance on occasion, and learning of the terrible circumstances in which the patients were treated caused her and others to feel "frantic to think that there is no equalization of material and of service, that there should be such a banking up in one place, and such desperate dearth in another."[45] This excess of labor and materials contrasted with the lack of experience and professionalism in the auxiliaries and led one English doctor to dismiss the care given at the hospital, commenting, "We do not trust our wounded to scented, painted ladies, or scented, painted men."[46] While La Motte was in good company with ninety-four other graduate nurses at the Ambulance, her perception of it as a place of excess and poor care eventually drove her to leave it and to look for other opportunities to nurse close to the front. In any case, her decision to publish "An American Nurse in Paris," laden with criticism about the excesses of the Ambulance, guaranteed that she would no longer be welcomed there once the piece was in print in July 1915.

La Motte's diary shows that by January 1915 she was no longer working at the hospital; she had only tolerated the atmosphere of excess for a very brief period. While she was amazed and frustrated by "the wastefulness of the institution,"[47] being free of the disproportionate luxuriousness of the hospital did not make finding a position in which she could use her skills and make a meaningful contribution to the war effort easier. As her diary reveals, her search ran into serious obstacles. The first attempt included an effort to travel with Giselle de Rancougne, the daughter of French engineer Philippe-Jean Bunau-Varilla, who was involved in the creation of the Panama Canal, and Madame Saanen-Algi, an American author who had written several books as Marie Louise Van Saanen, to the Western Front. The women, along with two American sculptors, Enid Yandell and Malvina Hoffman, had been involved in relief efforts, initiating the *Appui aux Artistes* to support artists and their families in August of 1914.[48] Yandell, whom La Motte had just met, recounted the story of a trip de Rancougne and Saanen-Algi had taken to the front where they saw wounded soldiers being treated in filthy conditions with only two nurses to care for several hundred wounded.[49] La Motte hoped to join de Rancougne and Saanen-Algi on their next trip to the front, but she was sorely disappointed when she could not get herself to Dunkirk, having no justification to obtain the necessary permission to travel to the war zone.

She would have to wait for another opportunity. One surfaced when she received an invitation from Mrs. Eleanor Sherman

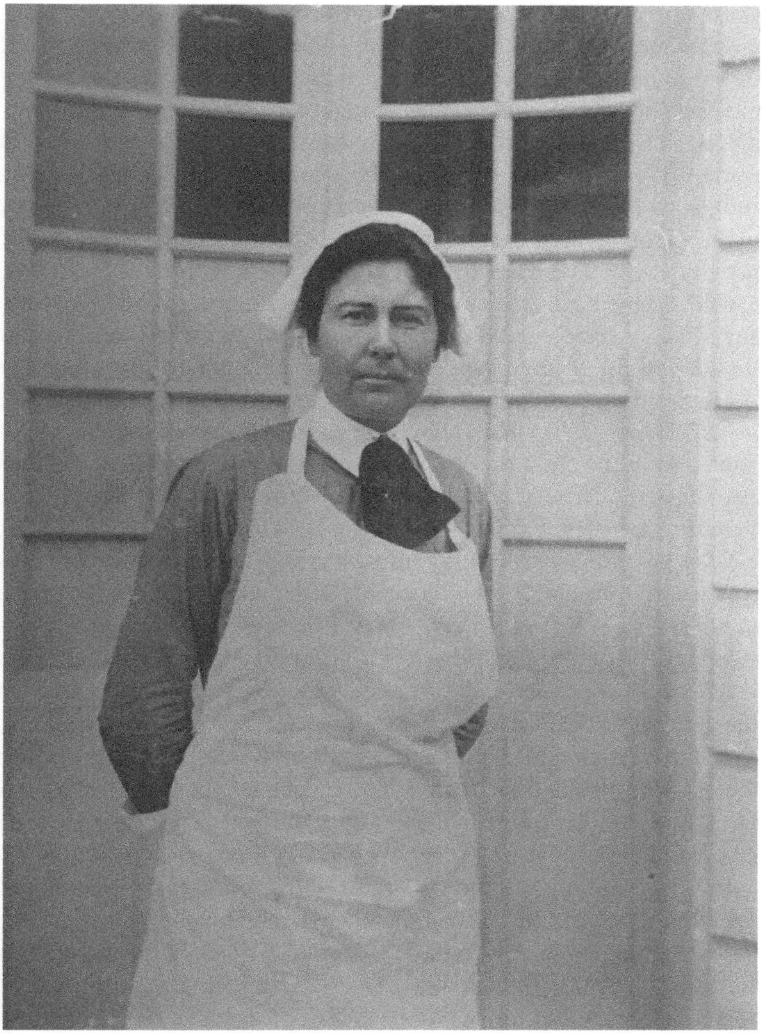

Figure 6 La Motte in nursing uniform, undated

Thackara, daughter of General William T. Sherman and wife of Alexander Thackara, the American Consul General at Paris, who had started a relief effort for the Serbian wounded. She reached out to La

Motte and invited her to take charge of the nurses in her unit traveling to Serbia. According to the *Sun*'s coverage of this development, La Motte had already left and was "giving her services to the famine and fever stricken Serbians."[50] In actuality, La Motte, though desperately seeking some kind of nursing position at or near the front, was hesitant if excited. Her diary describes going to see "G.S. this afternoon & to talk over the Serbian scheme with her."[51] Stein later wrote in *The Autobiography of Alice B. Toklas* that La Motte was "very heroic but gun shy,"[52] a comment which critics have often, perhaps unduly, noted.[53] Stein's brief assessment is only partially true. While La Motte was sensibly concerned about the dangers of the war zone, she did not allow those fears to paralyze her, and she mentions only one trip to see Stein and to discuss the Serbian expedition. La Motte made few comments in her diary about her apprehensions of nursing at the front, and in the end other pressures made the decision for her. After meeting with Thackara, she launched into a series of preparations, including sending a cable to her cousin, Alfred I. du Pont, asking "Shall I go to Serbia?"[54] His immediate and unequivocal reply was "Most certainly not."[55] At this point, in January of 1915, La Motte was in her early forties, an experienced professional nurse with years of being independent professionally and personally, yet her cousin's word effectively ended her prospects of going to Serbia. La Motte's diary doesn't make clear if she had to get permission from du Pont, or whether, as she did with Stein, La Motte wanted to mull over her choices with people she trusted, and since du Pont had long been a parental figure for La Motte ever since she had taken up residence with him in the fall of 1890,[56] it was logical for her to consult him.

La Motte did not question his refusal to grant her permission, but she felt a responsibility to complete what she had pledged to do for Thackara. She wrote in her diary, "I simply can't ditch the expedition so must at least take the nurses there, establish them, & then return."[57] In any case, the other nurses who were supposed to go received cables "forbidding them to go to Serbia!"[58] Despite this setback, she and Thackara decided the doctors would go ahead of the nurses and that La Motte would write a letter of appeal to du Pont "asking permission to take charge of [the expedition]"[59] so that the nurses could be organized to follow. She never discussed in the diary what du Pont's response was–in fact she never mentions him again in the diary–and never returned to the subject of the expedition. For whatever reason, the plan to get to the front through Thackara's connections did not come to fruition and La Motte turned her focus to seeking out other possible frontline nursing opportunities.

A month or so later La Motte refers to yet another tantalizing possibility of getting to the front with Saanen-Algi, who asked La Motte to visit her to discuss an opportunity, then never followed up on what must have been another disappointing failure to solidify a plan.[60] Her diary entries subsequently grew more sporadic, with as many as three weeks passing between them. According to the entries that she did make, La Motte's time was spent observing the country at war and lunching and dining with friends and acquaintances, including Stein and Toklas, with whom she waited out a zeppelin raid, accompanied by the Picassos, in the hallway of Stein's apartment building. The raid was followed by dinner with Stein and Toklas, during which the couple shared their plans to go to Spain to get away from the air raids.[61] Two days later La Motte reports that she and her friend Emily Chadbourne "raced around all day getting our papers for Spain."[62] Presumably they were to accompany Stein and Toklas on their trip south, but this plan too went awry when Chadbourne came down with "a bad tonsillitis" and La Motte observed, "This will knock out our trip to Spain, which we were to have set out on Monday night, for Barcelona."[63]

Other than a wistfulness in this brief line, La Motte expressed no thoughts of leaving for Spain without Chadbourne. Rather, she "got [her] directions from Dr. Austin" and "hurried back to Em," as she frequently called Chadbourne in the diary.[64] The nature of her relationship with Chadbourne at this point is ambiguous, though it is fair to assume that the two were in a relationship. Em, or E. C. as La Motte also referred to her, is mentioned with more frequency than anyone else in the diary, and as early as January 8, 1915, she describes having lunch with E. C. at Gertrude Stein's, the abbreviation of Chadbourne's name a sure indication of the familiarity between the two women. La Motte's decision to nurse Chadbourne points to their intimacy, but La Motte never discussed her with any particular warmth or affection, leaving the frequency of her interactions in the diary to suggest their closeness. How far back the friendship went is unclear. In a notarized letter attached to Chadbourne's 1916 passport application, La Motte asserted that she had known her "for a great many years," yet it is impossible to know if she was exaggerating the length of their acquaintanceship for legal purposes or if she really had known Chadbourne for a long time.[65]

Whatever the nature of their relationship in 1915, La Motte was devoted to Chadbourne and took on nursing her through her illness while still searching for an opportunity to get to the front. She was approached again about a possible war-related nursing opportunity when Gertrude Austin asked La Motte if she was interested in helping Countess van den Steen in Poperinge, Belgium with her "district nursing among the villagers, who are starving & destitute as well as ill."[66] This opportunity too came to naught and La Motte continued to fill her days with traveling to the Chateau de St. Lubin, which Chadbourne was considering buying, and making the social rounds with other Anglophones.

La Motte's frustrations, having accumulated since the start of the year at least, reached a peak when she received a letter from a cousin, Julia, communicating that "Lady Grogan, organizing the Expedition to Serbia, writes that she will be glad to see me, but can promise me nothing, as her list is an extremely long one already!"[67] This news provoked an exasperated outburst from La Motte: "That being so, I shan't go over to London to beg from a supercilious Englishwoman an opportunity to do hard work. All my altruism has now vanished. I'm not wanted, being a neutral. This is not our war, & there is no use in trying to force myself into a place."[68]

Just as La Motte was viewing the entire enterprise as hopeless, a friend, the journalist Paul Mowrer, contacted her. Mowrer was a foreign correspondent for the *Chicago Daily News*, a successful reporter who won acclaim for covering the war in the Balkans in 1912–1913 and then the war in Europe.[69] In her diary, La Motte mentions occasionally visiting the journalist and his first wife, Winifred Adams–he and Adams later divorced and Mowrer married Hadley Richardson Hemingway, Ernest Hemingway's first wife, in 1933–in the spring of 1915 before her departure for the war zone. She probably originally met him at gatherings at the Brasserie des Lilas, where, according to Theresa Helburn, Mowrer and his brother, Edgar, were "at the center of the group" that regularly gathered during the winter of 1913 and "were in touch with everything that was going on in Paris."[70] Though Helburn does not mention La Motte in her autobiography, she provided an affidavit swearing to La Motte's status as an American citizen,[71] and the two were friends. Helburn edited a draft of *The Tuberculosis Nurse* for La Motte and the two women probably attended the Mowrer gatherings together.[72] La Motte undoubtedly would have found them fascinating, given her interest in art and politics. By 1915, her friendship with the Mowrers was close enough that they gave her "a farewell 'demonstration'" at their apartment at 34, rue du Bac before her initial departure for Dunkirk.[73]

Mowrer helped to initiate the events that would eventually lead to her nursing at the front by delivering yet another tantalizing opportunity to pursue: an invitation to go and see John Borden, a friend of Mowrer's from Chicago, whose sister, Mary Turner,[74] was looking for nurses to staff her hospital.[75] La Motte immediately followed up on the suggestion and rushed over to meet him, but like all of the earlier opportunities that came within her grasp, this one eluded her when she discovered that John Borden had left Paris the same morning to return to the United States. What must have been keenly felt disappointment on La Motte's side turned into excitement when she was invited to meet with Mary Borden Turner on May 20 and learned that she had

> presented a portable hospital to the 8th Army Corps of France on condition that she could select the nurses. It consists of 8 [shacks], 6 for pts, holding 20 each. One for op & dressing rooms, & the 8th for kitchen & ourselves. It is to be set up at the rear of the lines, about 10 miles behind the firing line, which will be as far or farther forward than a field hospital is ever established. It can all be folded up & moved from place to place, & will follow the armies into Belgium or Germany![76]

Her final line joyously pronounced, "She accepted me!"[77]

La Motte immediately readied herself for service; she bought "French blouses & aprons, such as the Red Cross wear" on Turner's recommendation that it was more "tactful" to "wear the uniform the French Drs. are accustomed to."[78] In a rare moment of personal reflection, La Motte added, "My veil is pretty, but will be hard for a person like me to put on."[79] The meaning of this cryptic final line in that day's entry is ambiguous. La Motte may have been referring to the strangeness of dressing as a Red Cross nurse and the discomfort of putting on an unfamiliar nursing uniform. Her specific mention of the "veil" more likely suggests personal unease with such a feminine accessory. She was, according to all surviving photographic and documentary evidence, a woman who dressed simply. Whatever the source of her discomfort, La Motte quickly packed her bag, prepared to "travel as light as possible" and "ready to go any minute" after receiving notice from Borden Turner to leave.[80]

Getting to the front, however, would, in keeping with La Motte's months of waiting, take longer than anticipated. Borden Turner did not send word for La Motte to leave Paris until several weeks later. On June 20, with "E. C." accompanying her to the Gare du Nord train station, La Motte left for Dunkirk. The day before her departure she noted in a one-line paragraph, "I dread starting & uprooting myself."[81] She must have felt substantial apprehension at the uncertain future before her. During the first part of 1915 she had experienced Paris at war, including zeppelin raids, and engaged in battlefield tourism, visiting Senlis, a town less than thirty miles north of Paris, where she was guided by a man taken prisoner by German soldiers and then shot through the knee, and shown the wreckage of the town–the Germans had burned hundreds of houses in September 1914.[82] Several days later she traveled to Meaux, located twenty-five miles to the northeast of Paris, where the Germans had been stopped at the gates of the city during the First Battle of the Marne in September 1914. She describes seeing "graves in thousands every where, as far as the eye can reach–10,000 men are buried in the fields … Fearfully depressing these miles of graves."[83] Though she had dismissed the American Ambulance as a place of decadence and waste, when there she saw patients brought from the trenches, "dirty, muddy, bloody little heaps of humanity."[84] She describes the shock of seeing these men once their filthy clothes had been stripped and their wounds dressed by the doctor: "I saw the awful mutilation wrought by bullet and shrapnel."[85] While La Motte had undoubtedly seen injury, suffering, and death a great deal during her training and working life in Baltimore, this served as her first look at the effects of trench warfare on the human body. She quickly learned that "it is thus not so much the character of the wounds, terrible as these may be, but the resultant infections that lead to such disastrous consequences, and such serious and deforming mutilation."[86] In the diary, La Motte never connects these accumulated experiences to her anxiousness about what might be before her, but undoubtedly having some idea of the magnitude of the destruction of the war made her wary of the dangers and challenges that might lie ahead.

La Motte was also sensibly nervous about her own safety. Many nurses' narratives about war express indifference to the dangers they might have been in personally or they focus on their heroic efforts to protect their patients. A case in point is an anonymous work, *A War Nurse's Diary: Sketches from a Belgian Field Hospital*, published in 1918, in which the writer declares that "For some days the rumours were rife concerning the bombardment of Antwerp, but we did not take them seriously."[87] After the German bombardment begins, the nurse describes enduring it at close range, having refused the opportunity to return home to escape the inevitable occupation of the city by German forces. When she is frightened, her friend and fellow nurse reminds her, "Remember we are British women, not emotional continentals. We've got to keep our heads."[88] They seek shelter in a basement only to decide "that our place was beside our wounded."[89] They leave their shelter to help evacuate the wounded, placing themselves at significant risk as the city was heavily bombed and in a state of chaos. From her perspective, and one that is repeated in other nurses' narratives, part of her work as a nurse is to reflect the characteristics deemed to be part of the British national character: calm in the face of distress. Proving her loyalty to her patients was connected to ensuring she represented her nation well but was, more importantly, a professional duty that she willingly embraced. The tradition of depicting nurses as maternal beings ensured that nurses would feel a need to prove their devotion to their patients, for no woman abandons her children, especially when those children are in peril.

La Motte later witnessed a ceremony during which the brave actions of three nurses who stood by their patients during a bombardment were recognized: "a French general ... pinned the Croix de Guerre on the breast of each one, & kissed the hand of each. A very dignified & simple ceremony, but a ceremony & very moving!"[90] She clearly admired the nurses' actions and respected the attention bestowed on them as a result. In her own writing, she was more willing to share her fears about the dangers of the war zone, to which she was introduced very soon after her arrival in Malo, a small town near Dunkirk where she and other nurses were staying until Borden Turner's hospital was ready. Her diary entry for June 22 succinctly communicates being

"Waked at 2:45 a.m. by a bomb from a Taube."[91] La Motte and a nursing colleague ran outside to the beach in their pajamas to watch French airplanes in pursuit. She eventually returned to the hotel, only to go back out on the street at 5 a.m. to watch the shelling; she and several nurses later went into Dunkirk to rescue their supplies and found themselves under intense shelling. La Motte and her friend, Miss Irvine, eventually "Saw a woman enter a demolished house (previous bombardment) so ran & knocked. Man opened door, took us in cellar."[92] At no point in the entry does La Motte describe her own feelings as she wandered around an unfamiliar town under shell-fire. The most she says is "Were quite lost, did not know directions, no one in streets."[93] The end of the entry curtly reports "all to leave D. tomorrow for a few days, as hospital not ready till Saturday."[94]

La Motte sketched the bare bones of her experiences in the diary entry, saving a more prolonged and intense exploration of them for a published piece. In the article "Under Shell-Fire at Dunkirk," La Motte elaborates at some length on the feelings she was experiencing during the bombardment. In the article, she confesses to feeling a sense of being "locked in" upon entering "the war zone," an area only those with special permissions are allowed to enter.[95] As she observes, "Individual liberty was now gone; we were not free to come and go how and where we liked, but, under observation in the zone of the armies, we must share with the armies whatever fate had in store."[96] What that fate might be quickly became evident when she went out to explore Dunkirk, which by this time, "had been bombarded by long-range German guns,–siege guns fired from beyond Dixmunde, twenty-two miles away."[97] While the town buzzed with activity and townspeople conducting their everyday affairs, La Motte saw a "few ruined houses" and signs that people were preparing for the next possible attack by taping windows and putting up sandbags.[98] La Motte takes time to establish how this "day of glorious sunshine, of busy, homely occupation" is slowly pervaded by the sounds of guns, but the sounds seemed "so remote, so far away" that she goes to bed thinking, "this comfort and idleness might soon become a bore."[99]

That sense of security is shattered when bombs starting falling the next morning, driving her out to the beach, where hundreds of people are gathered to watch the Allies' planes in pursuit of the German Taubes. She does not yet feel afraid because she does "not know enough" and only finds the bombing "overwhelmingly interesting and exciting."[100] Her idle curiosity transforms into "a sickening sense of fear, of nervous dread" when she later ventures into Dunkirk to help remove some supplies at the docks to a safer place.[101] The town that she had so admired the previous day as people tranquilly went about their routine affairs is now "a scene of desolation and ruin."[102] Seeing "war in the concrete" and "the havoc wrought by those awful guns" increases her sense of dread and terror, which she internalizes, not revealing to her companion, "ever cheerful," the degree to which she was affected by the realization that she was "in Dunkirk, not after a bombardment, but between intervals of a bombardment!"[103] As she anticipated, the bombing starts anew, and La Motte describes what she had noted in abbreviated fashion in her diary: she and her companion desperately seek shelter. She, while fearfully looking for some way to get out of the open, realizes, "there was not one intellectual faculty I could call upon. There was nothing in past experience, nothing of will-power, of judgment, of intuition, that could serve me. I was beyond and outside and apart from the accumulated experience of a lifetime. My intelligence was worthless in this moment of supreme need."[104] At this point, La Motte was not a young woman unable to conceptualize mortal danger–as the narrator of *A War Nurse's Diary: Sketches from a Belgian Field Hospital* seems to be. Rather, she had seen the arbitrary nature of illness and injury during her long career as a nurse and fully realized the extreme danger she was exposed to while wandering the streets of Dunkirk. Not being able to use her experience and intellect to navigate the perils of her situation left her disoriented and uncomfortably vulnerable, both physically and emotionally.

They eventually hide in the basement of a building struck by a bomb two months earlier and now the underground dwelling place of a family that exhibited no reaction to the destruction of their home except for a "dignified acceptance of war."[105] When the bombing ceases and they know that the guns have to be left to cool before they will start firing again, La Motte and her companion leave their refuge and make an effort to return to their hotel in Malo, passing by "shattered houses; streets and sidewalks littered with broken glass, fallen bricks and rubbish; gaping walls open to the heavens."[106] They are rescued from this chaos when a truck picks them and takes them back to Malo. Once returned, La Motte describes the resumption of the bombing while they are eating lunch at their hotel. As it continues into the afternoon, the narrative perspective of the article shifts from past to present tense, locating the reader alongside her as she waits with the five other nurses, "calm, smiling, apparently indifferent" but feeling "a terrible tension as each shell falls."[107] Given that they have neither hospital nor patients to look after at this point, they have only their own welfare to consider. La Motte recognizes that "Should we desert now, take refuge in any of the ambulances that are below, that would so willingly carry us to a place of safety, the authorities would consider it an indication of how we would stand by our patients under fire."[108] Needing to prove her courage and loyalty to her profession, La Motte waits with the other nurses, smoking, eating chocolate, drinking coffee and tea, "writing … to kill time," and submitting to the realization that her survival is not contingent on any deliberate action she takes but on luck alone.[109]

Borden Turner was unwilling to trust to that luck and wanted the nurses to leave for Calais, where they would be safer. La Motte decided to continue on to Paris, where she stayed with "E. C." and resumed making rounds, lunching and dining out and attending the theater, for several days before returning to Malo on June 26. From there she went to Zuydcoote, a small Belgian town on the coast, staying at a hotel surrounded by a colonial regiment that attracted the attention of German Taubes. Her time in this small village was spent exploring the area, including a nearby sanitorium for tuberculosis patients, and visiting the hospital in Rousbrugge, where she was to take up her position. When she went to see it for the first time, "3 of the 13 shacks [were] up,"[110] an indication of the slow progress being made on the construction of the hospital. La Motte then moved to Rousbrugge on June 30, where she lodged at the *mairie* with several of the other nurses awaiting the opening of the hospital. This small, normally sleepy village was the "headquarters of the 8th Army, literally packed with soldiers & Belgian refugees."[111] From there she could smell a "stench like an abattoir" when the wind was blowing "straight from the battlefields."[112] Her stay was short-lived, however; when she visited the hospital she described it as "Well situated in a beautiful field, ¼ mile from village. 7 of 15 shacks are up, but no details finished in connection with them–will take 2 weeks more before they are ready."[113] With nothing to do but wait, La Motte traveled back to

Zuydcoote, where an Algerian regiment was encamped, leading one nurse to comment that they were "simply surrounded by savages!"[114] Her only other observation of colonial troops was to remark at the end of the same entry that "we heard one Arab committed suicide today."[115] She offers no speculation about why someone might make such a choice and never returns to this topic in her writing, though other incidents and themes from her diary are eventually worked into the sketches in *The Backwash of War*.

A theme La Motte explores in that collection is enclosure and stasis. La Motte described the sense of enclosure she originally felt after entering the war zone in her article "Under Shell-Fire" and in her diary, where she recorded, "Curious sensation of being shut in, in the war zone. One cannot go anywhere without papers–one cannot advance, retreat, or escape. Liberty is 0."[116] This nascent sentiment was amplified when she was forced to wait in Zuydcoote, initially surrounded by Algerians and then members of the Foreign Legion, which prompted her to observe, "We are going from bad to worse. All drinking heavily; cannot leave hotel, as dunes are full of them & beach is crowded with them, bathing. 3 were drowned this p.m. Bar full of soldiers, & others lying all round hotel, each with a bottle of wine."[117] La Motte's disgust at the Algerian regiment and the Foreign Legion unsurprisingly reflects the racist and classist attitudes evident in her work with the poor, immigrants, and African Americans discussed in Chapter 1. The revulsion she expresses also masks a fear of being vulnerable to the power the men around her wield. At the beginning of the day's entry, she recounts what happened to two nurses coming back late from Dunkirk: "[They] were held up by drunken sentry who put his bayonet to Waters' breast & threatened to shoot her."[118] Faced with physical threats, the women had no way to protect themselves and their only option was to take refuge in their rooms in hopes of going unnoticed.

La Motte's frustration with being enclosed increased as the precariousness of her situation became more evident the next day. A French fellow nurse, Mme. Raoul du Val, was stopped by a sentry who asked to see her *permis de séjour*. The nurses, however, had no official permission to be in the war zone. La Motte recalls having been told by Borden Turner that she did not need any–that she needed only to "say I belonged to her."[119] Borden Turner undoubtedly felt that her money and connections would be enough to vouch for the presence of the nurses in this restricted zone; the French authorities felt otherwise: Mme. Raoul du Val was informed that the nurses had "36 hours to get our papers in order, otherwise he would arrest us & send us to prison in D."[120] Borden Turner was away, leaving them without an authority figure to guide them. La Motte opined, "Very awkward to be left this way, at this [inaccessible] place. We have been virtual prisoners & now we are threatened in the actuality."[121] La Motte's feeling of being enclosed and deprived of her liberty was close to becoming a reality and she planned to return to Paris since she could not get a *permis de séjour* in Dunkirk because of her nationality. These obstacles and potential threats were wearing down her desire to serve, leading her to confess in her diary, "My enthusiasm for caring for wounded about vanished!"[122]

Mr. Burn, one of Borden Turner's drivers, agreed that their situation was "serious" and went to report it to Borden Turner, who had recently returned to Malo.[123] She was, according to La Motte's assessment, "looking thin & ill, & dreadfully upset over the departure of Col. Morier, who is being sent to the Front."[124] Morier was Borden Turner's ally and tried "to push things along, & with his departure the Ambulance will be left a prey to the opposition, jealousy, & hostility that everyone feels for it."[125] While La Motte was running into innumerable obstacles in her search for a nursing position, Borden Turner was doing the same on a larger scale as she tried to navigate the complexities of French military bureaucracy to keep the construction of the hospital on track.[126] Borden Turner decided La Motte should return to Paris, where she could get the paperwork she needed to stay in the war zone without fear of being arrested. From La Motte's perspective there was "No use waiting idle here–for even if we can walk about, it is intensely disagreeable by reason of the swarms of dirty, drunken soldiers that are all over the place. Spent our whole day indoors–the 3d in succession."[127] At this point, they were surrounded by an encamped "regiment of infantry–old men" for whom she felt no more compassion than she did for the Algerian regiment or the soldiers of the Foreign Legion.[128] La Motte perceived them all in the same negative light, their drunkenness encouraged by the policies of the French government. She learned from the owner of their hotel that "the Govt. will not permit him to sell spirits to soldiers but he has carte blanche to sell them as much wine as they can hold."[129] La Motte left for Paris the next day. She escaped the confines of the war zone and spent more than a week in Paris, staying with "E. C.," "who took [her] in" when she arrived late on the night of July 6.[130]

Though La Motte left much of this week in Paris undocumented in her diary, she did discuss completing a series of errands given to her by Borden Turner and resuming her life in Paris, going to the *Comédie Française* and sharing meals with various friends, often in the company of Chadbourne. She visited Mowrer to get feedback on an article she had written. While he was fourteen years younger than La Motte, she recognized his talent–he eventually won a Pulitzer Prize in 1929–and sought out his professional opinion regarding her work. She does not name the piece she took to him in July, but Mowrer liked it and said "it [was] dramatically done."[131] In all likelihood it was "Under Shell-Fire at Dunkirk," which was eventually printed in the fall of 1915 in the *Atlantic Monthly*, the first time La Motte was published in this widely read magazine, giving her the opportunity to reach a more varied audience than she previously had with her writings about nursing and suffrage.

When La Motte took the train to Dunkirk on the morning of July 16, she would not return to Paris until three months later. In July, she would finally do the kind of useful nursing work she had been yearning to do since the previous August. The long-drawn-out process of getting to the front undoubtedly heightened her nervousness about her departure, and the night before leaving she was filled with longing for home and not anticipation of the challenges in front of her. After spending a day busily running errands and meeting with a variety of people for lunch, tea, and dinner, she remarks: "Felt very homesick tonight. Wish the war was over, & that I could go back to America. They don't like us here–it's not our country, & now that we aren't over here, spending money right & left, they make no disguise of their real feelings."[132] Her comments underline her resentment at what she perceives as the greediness of the French and their dislike of Americans and present something of a conundrum: how is she to work in a hospital under the control of the French and provide compassionate care to French patients while feeling so much antipathy for them? Undoubtedly her apprehension at returning to the war zone with its attendant dangers and the uncertainties about her nursing position were increasing her anxiety and heightening her feelings of bitterness about the French. Her ability to care for and work with the French and to manage her own anxieties would soon be put to the test as she finally, after more than half a year of searching, assumed her nursing position at *L'Hôpital Chirurgical Mobile No. 1.*

Notes

1 "No Faith in Militancy," *Sun* (August 12, 1914), p. 3.
2 "News Notes," *JHNAM* 9:3 (July 1914), p. 109.
3 Records show she moved to 166 boulevard Montparnasse, Paris in September 1913 "for the purpose of study." National Archives and Records Administration, Washington, DC (hereafter NARA), General Records of the Department of State, 1763–2002, Record Group 59, Consular Registration Certificates, Compiled 1907–1918, ARC ID: 1244186.
4 The *JHNAM* notes that her book was almost finished by then. See "News Notes," *JHNAM* 13:3 (July 1914), p. 109. La Motte discusses completing a draft in April, being almost done with revisions in May, and having sent it to the USA in June. See JHMI, Ellen N. La Motte Collection, "La Motte to Amy Wesselhoeft von Erdberg," April 11, 1914, May 6, 1914, and June 11, 1914. A letter of acknowledgement of receipt of the manuscript shows that G. P. Putnam's Sons had the manuscript by early October. Private Collection, "G. P. Putnam's Sons to Ellen La Motte," October 8, 1914.
5 JHMI, "La Motte to Wesselhoeft von Erdberg," October 31, 1913.
6 JHMI, "La Motte to Wesselhoeft von Erdberg," November 22, 1913.
7 *Ibid.*
8 JHMI, "La Motte to Wesselhoeft von Erdberg," December 25, 1913.
9 Private Collection, Ellen N. La Motte, *Drafts of Unfinished Stories and Sketches, 1911–1919* (hereafter *Drafts*), "Les Transatlantiques."
10 For a discussion of Stein and her circle in Paris, see James R. Mello, *Charmed Circle: Gertrude Stein and Company* (New York: Henry Holt, 1974) and Shari Benstock, "Gertrude Stein and Alice B. Toklas: Rue de Fleurus," in *Women of the Left Bank: Paris, 1900–1940* (Austin, TX: University of Texas Press, 1986), pp. 143–193.
11 JHMI, "La Motte to Wesselhoeft von Erdberg," October 31, 1913.
12 Margaret R. Higonnet asserts that the two did know each other in Baltimore. See "Introduction," in *Nurses at the Front* (Boston: Northeastern University Press, 2001), p. xi.
13 Private Collection, Ellen N. La Motte, Unpublished Diary (hereafter Diary), "January 7, 1915."

14 *Ibid.*, "January 14, 1915." La Motte noted in the diary that this entry should be for January 8.
15 JHMI, "La Motte to Wesselhoeft von Erdberg," October 31, 1913.
16 Margaret R. Higonnet theorizes the impact of cubism, as La Motte would have been exposed to it through visits to Stein's apartment, in "Cubist Vision in Nursing Accounts," in *First World War Nursing: New Perspectives*, ed. Alison S. Fell and Christine E. Hallett (Abingdon: Routledge, 2013), pp. 156–172.
17 JHMI, "La Motte to Wesselhoeft von Erdberg," April 11, 1914.
18 For more information about the Clapps and their relationship with La Motte, see Chapter 4.
19 JHMI, "La Motte to Wesselhoeft von Erdberg," May 6, 1914.
20 JHMI, "La Motte to Wesselhoeft von Erdberg," April 29, 1915.
21 See Chapter 1, n. 64, for more information about Lent.
22 La Motte, *Drafts*, "The Flea Fair."
23 *Ibid.*
24 La Motte, *Drafts*, "Petria Smolianinoff."
25 La Motte, *Drafts*, "Les Transatlantiques."
26 *Ibid.*
27 *Ibid.*
28 For discussion of Louise and her relationship with La Motte, see Chapter 2.
29 JHMI, "La Motte to Wesselhoeft von Erdberg," December 23, 1911.
30 *Ibid.*
31 La Motte, *Drafts*, "By-Products."
32 *Ibid.*
33 La Motte, Diary, "January 7, 1915."
34 See Chapter 1 for a discussion of La Motte's tuberculosis nursing career.
35 La Motte, Diary, "January 19, 1915."
36 Ellen N. La Motte, "An American Nurse in Paris," *Survey* 34:15 (July 1915), p. 333. Various critics, including most recently Hazel Hutchison, in *The War that Used Up Words: American Writers and the First World War* (New Haven, CT: Yale University Press, 2015), p. 141, logically suggest that Gertrude Stein was probably the one to send the message to La Motte. It was, however, Gertrude Austin. As recorded in La Motte's diary, she frequently met with Dr. and Mrs. Austin from January through July 1915. Dr. Austin (1857–1938) was Cecil Kent Austin. He was born in Chicago, earned his B.A. from Yale, trained at the Paris Faculty of Medicine, and in 1915 had been practicing medicine in France for twenty-five years. See *Bulletin of Yale University: Obituary Records of Graduates of Yale University Deceased during the Year 1938–1939* 36 (January 1940), p. 25. He married Ellen Gertrude Binney in 1895. According to entries in La Motte's diary, she was involved in the French Flag Nursing Corps. See La Motte, Diary, "June 8, 1915." Later, Mrs. Austin headed up the Surgical Dressings Service Department of the American National Red Cross. See "Red Cross Pushed Co-Operative Plan," *New York Times*, August 6, 1917, p. 16.

37 Frederick Mortimer Clapp Papers (hereafter FMCP), Yale Collection of American Literature, Beinecke Rare Book and Manuscript Library, New Haven, CT, "Gertrude Austin to Ellen La Motte," October 6, 1914.
38 "News Notes," *JHNAM* 13:4 (October 1914), p. 214.
39 La Motte, "An American Nurse," p. 333.
40 *Ibid.*
41 *Ibid.*
42 *Ibid.*
43 *Ibid.*, p. 335.
44 *Ibid.*
45 *Ibid.*
46 *Ibid.*
47 *Ibid.*, p. 334.
48 "Americans Aid French Artists," *New York Times*, 30 May 1915, p. SM20.
49 La Motte, Diary, "January 4, 1915."
50 "Work Too Easy in Paris," *Sun* (July 11, 1915), p. 4.
51 La Motte, Diary, "January 18, 1915."
52 Gertrude Stein, *The Autobiography of Alice B. Toklas* (New York: Vintage, 1990), p. 158.
53 For example, see Higonnet, "Introduction," pp. xi and xiii, and Hutchison, *The War that Used Up Words*, p. 141.
54 La Motte, Diary, "January 24, 1915."
55 *Ibid.*
56 See the Introduction for a discussion of La Motte's use of the term father in relation to du Pont.
57 La Motte, Diary, "January 24, 1915."
58 *Ibid.*, "January 25, 1915."
59 *Ibid.*
60 *Ibid.*, "March 1, 1915."
61 *Ibid.*, "March 25, 1915."
62 *Ibid.*, "March 27, 1915."
63 *Ibid.*, "March 28, 1915."
64 *Ibid.*
65 See the Introduction for more discussion of the nature of La Motte and Chadbourne's relationship. NARA, Passport Applications for Travel to China, 1906–1925, Box 4424, Volume 12, "Emergency Passport Applications: China."
66 La Motte, Diary, "April 1, 1915." Countess van den Steen was heavily involved in relief work for civilians in Belgium for the duration of the war. See P. U. Kellogg, *The Fourth Year in Belgium: How Help is Reaching the Lowlands through the American Red Cross* (Washington, DC: American Red Cross, 1918), p. 16.
67 La Motte, Diary, "May 3, 1915."
68 *Ibid.*

69 For more information about Mowrer see the Paul Scott Mowrer Papers, The Newberry Library, Chicago. The only trace of La Motte in his papers is her name and address, and those of Chadbourne, scrawled haphazardly in an address book in the collection.
70 Theresa Helburn, *A Wayward Quest: The Autobiography of Theresa Helburn* (Boston: Little, Brown, and Company, 1960), p. 31.
71 NARA, General Records of the Department of State, 1763–2002, Record Group 59, Consular Registration Certificates, Compiled 1907–1918.
72 JHMI, "La Motte to Wesselhoeft von Erdberg," April 11, 1914.
73 La Motte, Diary, "May 27, 1915."
74 La Motte always refers to Mary Borden Turner by her married name, "Mrs. Turner," in the diary. Borden divorced her first husband, Douglas Turner, in 1918 and immediately married Edward Spears. She published most of her books under the name Mary Borden and is usually referred to as such by scholars. For the sake of clarity, I refer to her as Borden Turner. For more information about her life, see Jane Conway, *A Woman of Two Wars: The Life of Mary Borden* (London: Munday, 2010).
75 La Motte, Diary, "May 9, 1915."
76 *Ibid.*, "May 20, 1915."
77 *Ibid.*
78 *Ibid.*, "May 24, 1915."
79 *Ibid.*
80 *Ibid.*, "May 25, 1915."
81 *Ibid.*, "June 19, 1915."
82 *Ibid.*, "May 5, 1915."
83 *Ibid.*, "May 8, 1915."
84 La Motte, "An American Nurse," p. 333.
85 *Ibid.*, p. 334.
86 *Ibid.*
87 Anonymous, *A War Nurse's Diary: Sketches from a Belgian Field Hospital* (New York: Macmillan, 1908), p. 19.
88 *Ibid.*, p. 22.
89 *Ibid.*
90 La Motte, Diary, "July 23, 1915."
91 *Ibid.*, "June 22, 1915."
92 *Ibid.*
93 *Ibid.*
94 *Ibid.*
95 Ellen N. La Motte, "Under Shell-Fire at Dunkirk," *Atlantic Monthly* (November 1915), p. 692.
96 *Ibid.*
97 *Ibid.*, p. 693.
98 *Ibid.*

99 *Ibid.*, pp. 693–694.
100 *Ibid.*, p. 695.
101 *Ibid.*, p. 696.
102 *Ibid.*
103 *Ibid.*, pp. 696–697.
104 *Ibid.*, p. 698.
105 *Ibid.*, p. 699.
106 *Ibid.*
107 *Ibid.*, p. 700.
108 *Ibid.*
109 Hazel Hutchison offers a reading of La Motte's description of herself writing as a way for La Motte to defy death and defend "the cultural worth of text." See Hutchison, *The War that Used Up Words*, p. 147.
110 La Motte, Diary, "June 28, 1915."
111 *Ibid.*, "June 30, 1915."
112 *Ibid.*, "July 1, 1915."
113 *Ibid.*
114 *Ibid.*
115 *Ibid.*, "July 2, 1915."
116 *Ibid.*, "June 20, 1915."
117 *Ibid.*, "July 3, 1915."
118 *Ibid.*
119 *Ibid.*, "July 4, 1915."
120 *Ibid.*
121 *Ibid.*
122 *Ibid.*
123 *Ibid.*, "July 5, 1915."
124 *Ibid.*
125 *Ibid.* Morier was also Borden Turner's lover for a time. See La Motte, Diary, "September 15–16, 1915."
126 See Conway, *A Woman of Two Wars*, especially chs 3 and 4, for an overview of Borden Turner's struggle to set up and run the hospital.
127 La Motte, Diary, "July 5, 1915."
128 *Ibid.*
129 *Ibid.*
130 *Ibid.*, "July 6, 1915."
131 *Ibid.*, "July 15, 1915."
132 *Ibid.*

4

At the frontlines, 1915–1916

La Motte's search to put her nursing expertise to use found satisfaction when she was taken on by Borden Turner; however, instead of feeling fulfilled at long last by the expectation of helping the wounded with her excellent skills and extensive experience as a nurse, she encountered a myriad of vexations brought on by different nursing standards and cultural differences. The frustrations accumulated during six months of searching for war work would be compounded by the realities of working in what she saw as "neither a base nor a field hospital. A field would lay no emphasis on niceties & luxuries–a base would be better staffed."[1] Her diary, kept with regularity from the time she arrived at the hospital until her departure in early October 1915, which marked the end of the first of three trips to the hospital, aligns with nursing historian Christine Hallett's assertion that "trained nurses were more likely to write about what they did than about how they felt."[2] At least, with regard to her patients and the work she did for them, La Motte rarely provided details, preferring to sketch her work in broad strokes except when clinically describing some of her patients' wounds.[3] She expresses occasional empathy for some of the suffering she witnessed, but the rest of the emotions recorded in the diary are derived from her anger at being both overworked and underutilized in the hospital and her dismay at what she viewed as poor treatment of the patients.

It would not take long after her arrival in the war zone for these aggravations to begin accumulating. La Motte was quickly sent to Rousbrugge, where she had her first look at the hospital as it approached a state of completion. Her reaction was positive: "our hospital–Ambulance Chirurgical No. 1; Whole place looks very

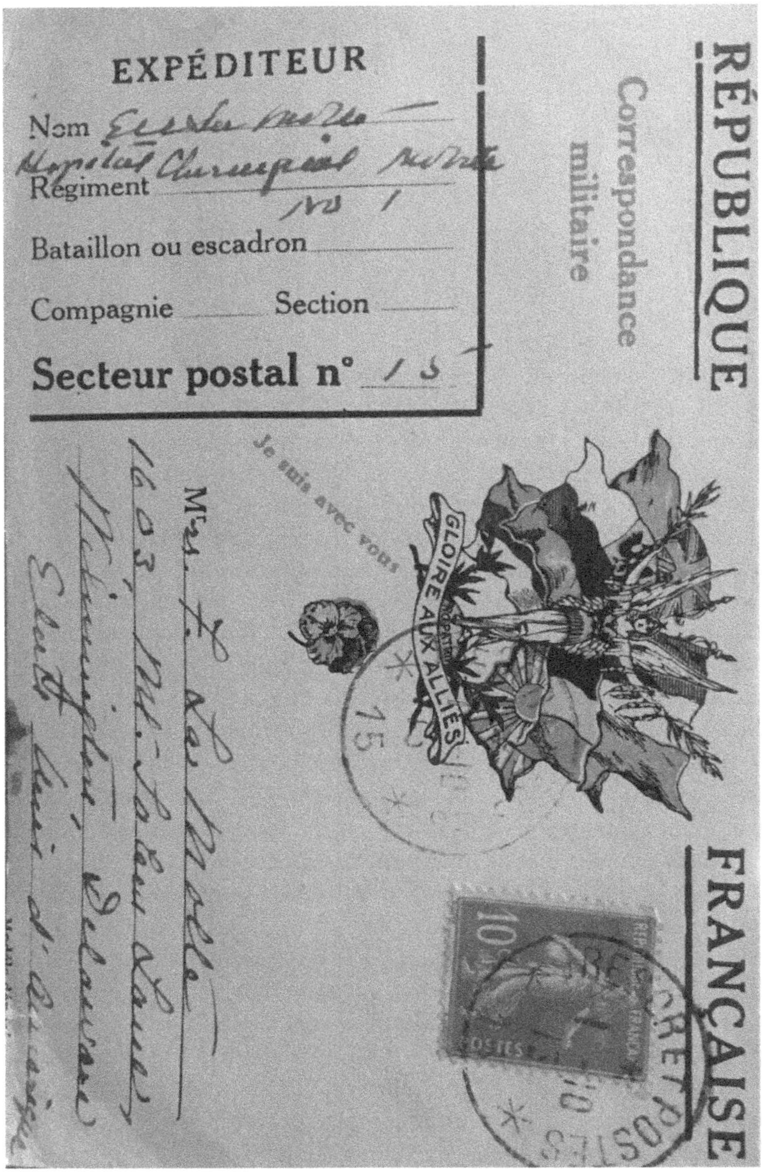

Figure 7 Postcard from La Motte from *L'Hôpital Chirurgical Mobile No. 1* to her mother in Wilmington, DE

nice–15 or so wooden barraques or huts, arranged sequentially on a field connected by board walks. There are seven wards of [?] beds, an O.R.–X-ray rooms; kitchen & laundry; pharmacy & waiting or receiving room; linen & supply room; Drs hut; nurses hut, & bureau for Mrs. Turner."[4] She communicates a sense of optimism and pride at being part of a new and well-organized hospital.[5]

Riding on that initial energy, she immediately set about making her living space in a section of the nurses' hut more hospitable by putting up a shelf and improvised washstand made of a packing crate. She then went to work with the other nurses, dismantling iron beds and carrying them and their supply of linen to different huts. La Motte does not complain about doing what must have been physically tiring work for her, given that she was many years from the days when she did heavy nursing, but she does make arch observations about the French doctors and orderlies: "The doctors looked at us struggling along with the heavy beds, but never offered to lend a hand. We have 38 *infirmiers* but this is Sunday, their day off, so they sat on the grass playing cards & watching us."[6] Very probably, the doctors and orderlies were confounded by these women, some of whom, like La Motte, were highly trained professional nurses, working so close to the front. The French had few such nurses at the beginning of the war and officially, if not in practice, barred female nurses from the war zone until spring 1917.[7] La Motte's early observation is the first of many that she would make in the diary about the behavior of the French medical staff. If La Motte disliked their unprofessional behavior, the French resented the presence of foreigners in the hospital, as attested to when a French general came to came to visit the hospital. La Motte reported that "word was sent for us all to hide ourselves as the Gen. hates us all, & we were not to irritate him by our presence. The French people certainly resent our being here, yet they never fail to squeeze [?] out of Mrs. T. at every turn. It is too damnable!"[8]

While the French came under her critical eye, they were not the only ones. An issue La Motte struggled with during her time at the hospital was the amateurism of some of the women working with her. The process of setting up the hospital was slowed by insufficient supplies and, at least from La Motte's perspective, the fact that "There is no professional head in the place, so we take orders & are directed by an amateur–Mrs. Abraham. She is awfully nice, but simply doesn't know."[9] Mrs. Abraham, whose husband was serving in the military and used to come by to visit her on occasion, was Borden Turner's English friend, and, like her, had no professional training as a nurse. La Motte's patience, already thin to begin with, was tested by working with people who did not meet her professional standards. In addition, the close proximity in which the nurses had to live and work exacerbated an already trying situation, and she recorded that on only their second day of working together, "Off and on all day we hear the guns, but it is remote. The noise of our work & talk drowns them. Very quiet & peaceful here. We all sit about together & discuss how we can best screen off our rooms, to get away from each other."[10] While the hospital environment was currently "quiet" and "peaceful," this would not last much longer. Soon the hospital began accepting patients and the tensions between the nurses became more strained as they had to learn to navigate their cultural and professional differences as they began the business of caring for their patients.

Despite having spent many long months and having overcome many obstacles while waiting to nurse the wounded, La Motte observed the arrival of the first patients at the hospital on July 24, 1915 with less attention to detail and excitement than might be expected. She devoted only a few lines of that day's diary entry to the experience: "At 4 p.m. our first pt. arrived–[knee] shattered by a shell. My work in the receiving ward went off smoothly. Later, at 7 p.m. another case was brought in, a shoulder, a delay of only 6 hrs. in each case, from the time of injury, till in our hands. All frightfully excited & interested over our farm yard & our first wounded."[11] The farmyard to which she is referring received more diary space on that day than the arrival of the wounded. She and several of the French nurses decided to buy a pig, cock, hen, ducks, and a kid, which she named Esmeralda,[12] to help create "an air of cheerfulness & hominess to the hospital, 10 miles from the Front!"[13]

The rate at which patients arrived at the hospital remained a dribble for some time. The slow pace allowed for the nurses to adjust to receiving the wounded and gave time for La Motte to assess coolly the nursing abilities of the others. La Motte, undoubtedly because of her experience and competence, was immediately put in charge of *Salle II* as well as the *Salle des Entrées*. She shared duty hours with Mlle. Morin, whom she rather condescendingly described as "a nice little Fr. woman, who knows surgical technique, but nothing about nursing."[14] Other nurses fell apart under the strain of caring for even a few patients; La Motte describes what happened to one English nurse: "Poor Waters, who was on night duty last night, lost her nerve & went to pieces. Has been taken off hospital work & put in charge of the linen room."[15] There undoubtedly had to be some embarrassment and shame attached to being unable to handle the rigors of nursing, and La Motte did not hesitate to pass judgment, at least in the privacy of her diary, on those who did not have the skills and wherewithal to withstand them. She saved her most virulent criticism, however, for another French nurse, Leclerc, about whom she commented: "Had a trying day today. Was put in charge of *Salle III*, with one of the *Croix de Guerre* nurses, Leclerc. An insufferable idler, & an insidious, dangerous woman, who is going to make trouble, if she can between French & English, & their methods of nursing."[16] The next day she reported her most withering assessment: that Leclerc was "ignorant & common & no more of a nurse than 'Esmeralda.' "[17] La Motte does not say what Leclerc did that so earned her enmity, but La Motte's position in relation to many of the nurses would remain unrelentingly critical and constitute a serious source of stress for her during these early months of work.

The source of much of her anxiety lay in the assumptions La Motte brought about nursing care and quality. Hallett claims that La Motte "was probably one of the most highly trained nurses of her generation,"[18] yet she had to work in a milieu where there were contrasting understandings of what a nurse was and little appreciation for the immense ability she could put into action. During the war in France the term "nurse" did not designate one kind of trained professional; rather, the word could be used to refer to trained and untrained men and women with varying degrees of expertise and experience.[19] By mid-1915, when La Motte went to work in Belgium, many French nurses might possess a training certificate received through the French Red Cross after a brief three-month course or nursing duties might be carried out by *infirmiers* (orderlies) with very little training or experience who were not subject to the authority of the more experienced nurses on the wards. After the 1907 decision by the French Ministry of War to allow lay women to be assigned to military hospitals, it was established that they would not serve at or near the frontlines–that restriction would be lifted in 1917, though as La Motte's practical experience shows, female nurses were providing care in close proximity to the trenches much earlier in the war.[20] At the same time, it was determined that medical students and male nurses would provide most of the patient care and female nurses would do "domestic work," such as giving patients their meals.[21] Based on this understanding of nursing, it is not surprising that a three-month certificate was viewed as adequately preparing women for hospital nursing.

The dire nature of wartime casualties would, however, through necessity, eventually redefine some of ways in which female nurses would be used in military hospitals. La Motte, working in the early years of the war, struggled to contend with working with uneven and unqualified assistance. A month into her nursing work, she expressed her upset with the French orderlies–those who were supposed to offer more substantial and valuable care than she was:

> Do hate this feeling of "getting on" with my orderlies. They are all on my professional level, in the eyes of the Service de Santé, & it is [enraging] to get what little I get, by wheedling & being decent. Sergeant [?], the head, always makes rounds with the Drs & takes their orders, & Rouhier explains fully to [?] what he wants in the way of diet. [?] gives the medicines, etc–it all goes through him. I give piqures & serums, but doubtless [?] could do it as well. The Santé has no idea of nursing care, & these orderlies, strong young men, who ought to be in the trenches, are shirking work doing women's jobs. I have 6 on my ward–6 for 11 pts. With one good nurse as [*sic*] one good orderly, the work could be better done. Many orderlies impudent to the nurses. Mine are not as I never insist on their doing something that they will refuse to do. We get on amiably, but I hate my deference towards [?], my overlooking of so much in the others.[22]

Her frustrations with her orderlies, untrained, undisciplined, and not subordinate to her in any way, echoes the confusion that many British and American trained nurses operated in when they volunteered in French military hospitals.[23]

The conflicts in the hospital, ignited by differing concepts regarding the kind and quality of care patients needed, came to a head when Borden Turner decided to file charges against a Dr. Bordeau. She was driven to do so when a patient was left "soaked in blood all night" because the doctor refused to attend to him even after being called repeatedly by Borden Turner.[24] Bordeau claimed to be sick, yet he refused to give his patient to one of the other doctors. The reasons for his obstinacy were never identified, though La Motte believed he was "indifferent" despite the fact the patient was suffering from a "gas infection."[25] The doctor's negligence enraged Borden Turner, who immediately reported him to his superiors and threatened to close down the hospital if he were not let go. There was an inquiry the next day, when a general from the *Service de santé* arrived to hear her accusations and the doctor's rebuttal. According to La Motte, Borden Turner was a "wreck" after the proceedings, fearing that her ultimatum would be accepted.[26] Three days later the struggle for control over the hospital was resolved when Borden Turner was castigated by the general from the *Service the santé* for her lack of medical knowledge and for having brought charges that could ruin the doctor's career.[27] The general also advised her that had she asked for him to be transferred without bringing charges, this could have been done, allowing all of them to save face and the doctor his career. She took this scolding badly and wanted to resign "since she has no authority & cannot insist of [*sic*] a high standard of work."[28]

La Motte's reflections on the doctor's behavior and Borden Turner's subsequent actions were more sanguine. She wrote:

> Most of the day spent in long conversations. The gist of the matter is this: Mrs. T. was allowed to establish this hospital through the influence of Col. Morier. It was neither wanted not [*sic*] needed. She asked to have it under military control & failed to realize that the gift once accepted, the [?] between the gift, & the giver would widen every day. Under military control she has absolutely nothing to say as to its management, but must stand by & accept & be unable to remedy any mismanagement that may take place. The question is, is she willing to keep her ideals, & give up the work when she can't realize them, or is she going to compromise, to accept French standards, & do the best she can with them. The cynical attitude of the French nation on the subject of health & hospitals, & their antique methods of dealing with illness, are something she ought to reconcile herself with if she stays. Gross neglect of a pt. occurred here; she was unable to remedy that–she sent a letter saying she would leave if things were not altered–things were not altered, she was called a capricious child–and she stays.[29]

La Motte, trained in a hierarchical system at Johns Hopkins and used to working in a bureaucracy from her days at the Health Department in Baltimore, was much more resigned to the structure of the hospital and wavered between compassion for Borden Turner's frustrations and exasperation with her unrealistic ideals.

The next day, the tension was lessened when Borden Turner left the hospital "to spend a few days with her husband & children."[30] La Motte observed that "the relief of her departure, relief from the [trouble] we have all been under, is very marked. I rather enjoyed my ward tonight for the first time."[31] She continued her musings about Borden Turner's role in the hospital and her restlessness: "Mrs. T. getting back her balance again, but the truth is, she is dreadfully bored. As 'Directrice' her title is out of courtesy, she is simply head of the nursing staff, which was all I ever thought she expected to be. She is frankly bored with the whole thing, now that her ideals of attaining perfecti[on] have been clipped in the bud."[32] An increase in patients and activity in the hospital coincided with Borden Turner's absence, but La Motte did not miss her and remarked, "Great relief having Mrs. T. off the place with all these terribly wounded men."[33]

These wounded men began to occupy more space in La Motte's diary, and La Motte started to record her observations of her patients more fully, including details that would eventually make their way into the sketches included in *The Backwash of War*. One of her first patients, a transfer from another hospital, "had tried to kill himself in June–shot himself, the ball wounding his foot. Has been a [prisoner] ever since, & is to be tried shortly for desertion, & if not acquitted, will be shot. A poor, fragile weak man, so grateful for a bath & the comfort we gave him–he was afraid of the trenches & tried to end it the other way–and failed. Eugene [C—] his name–44 yrs old–a reservist."[34] More than a month later, she recorded that on a very busy day on her ward, which she described as "a perfect hell," a "man [was] brought in who tried to commit suicide. Shot himself through the mouth–fearful sight. Saw them as they began to operate. Rouhier says why should anyone attempt suicide these days, when it is so easy to obtain death with honor right at hand."[35]

These two entries combined contain the seeds of the first story she published about nursing in a frontline hospital, "Heroes." The piece was originally published in the *Atlantic Monthly* in August of 1916 and later served as the opening story of *The Backwash of War*. While the *Atlantic Monthly* had begun publishing stories and articles under a separate section titled "The Great War" in February 1916, and in August 1916 published five pieces clustered under that heading, "Heroes" was wedged between "The Odyssey of the Sockeye Salmon" and "A Federal Merchant Marine" in the main body of the issue, suggesting that the editors did not perceive this short piece of fiction as meshing with the non-fiction pieces exploring the war experience, and written by men, clustered in the separate section. Another piece by her, "A Joy Ride," published two months later, was not placed in the Great War section either, though Maud Mortimer Clapp's "Behind the Yser," published in the same issue, was. Clapp's story forms part of her longer work, *A Green Tent in Flanders*, released by Doubleday, Page & Company in 1917.[36] The book consists of a series of sketches derived from Clapp's time at *L'Hôpital Chirurgical Mobile No. 1*, a position that La Motte helped her to obtain. While the two were once friends, by the time they finished working together in the hospital, Clapp loathed La Motte and wrote her book as a deliberate refutation of the view of the war presented in La Motte's *The Backwash of War*.

What Clapp and other readers of La Motte's writings about World War One found objectionable was its unadorned view of her patients. She refused to idealize them and their suffering and frequently focused on the degradation of humans caught in extreme circumstances. In "Heroes," for example, the story opens with a troubling description of one soldier's desperation:

> When he could stand it no longer, he fired a revolver up through the roof of his mouth, but he made a mess of it … so they bundled him into an ambulance and carried him, cursing and screaming, to the nearest field hospital …. To save his life he must reach the hospital without delay … He was a deserter, and discipline must be maintained. Since he had failed in the job, his life must be saved; he must be nursed back to health, until he was well enough to be stood up against a wall and shot.[37]

This gruesome initial paragraph undermines wartime ideals such as glory, heroism, and courage while questioning the way in which she, as a nurse, perpetuates this system. The reader might expect the pointlessness of nursing a man destined to die by firing squad to be contrasted with the meaningfulness of saving other more worthy soldiers; however, the narrator of the story finds no such consolation. Instead, she interrogates the meaning of her nursing efforts when she ponders:

> His mind [the suicide's] seemed fixed on death .... He was so different from the other patients, who wanted to live. It was a joy to nurse them .... By expert surgery, by expert nursing, some of these were to be returned to their homes again, *réformés*, mutilated for life, a burden to themselves and to society; others were to be nursed back to health, to a point at which they could again shoulder eighty pounds of marching kit, and be torn to pieces again on the firing line. It was a pleasure to nurse such as these.[38]

Whatever the reason for the injury, a self-inflicted wound or one received from the enemy, the end result is the same: more exposure to potential death or a trip home with serious bodily injury. Rather than perceiving herself as a healer, or a saver of lives, the narrator sees her professional self as an integral part of the cyclical motion of war, condemning nurses for their complicity and denouncing the entire military structure.

By late August 1915, when the hospital was busy and La Motte was feeling exhausted by the pace of work, she had come to share her narrator's questioning of the meaning and purpose of nursing those destined to die. Her physical fatigue was undoubtedly exacerbated by her inability to believe in the nobility of their mission. She explains in a letter to Clapp from the end of August, "it seems such an ironic waste of time–to patch up the men who go back to be killed, & to patch up & prolong the lives & suffering of those who would better be dead. Your hopeful cases go back to be shot at, & your hopeless ones you 'save' in order to burden society with wastage & wreck. Is aiding & abetting this an actual thing to do? Now don't be mushy & sentimental, and be honest & stripped bare, that's what your ministering angel does."[39] La Motte's stark understanding of nursing in wartime found release in her creative writing, in which she dissected the system that supported this, in her eyes, pointless cycle. For example, in "Heroes," her narrator does not censure the man who has attempted to kill himself; rather, she critiques the system that would drive a man to end his life. When the doctors and nurses are trying to administer ether, she comments:

> [I]t was very difficult to get the man under the anæsthetic. Many cans of ether were used, which went to prove that the patient was a drinking man. Whether he had acquired the habit of hard drink before or since the war could not be ascertained; the war had lasted a year now, and in that time many habits may be formed.[40]

The narrator recognizes that the stress of combat and the inhumanity of the trenches lead men to any means of escape, including alcoholism and suicide. While she depicts this one soldier in a less than idealized light, the narrator passes judgment on the other soldiers in her care as well. She compares the suicidal soldier to the rest of the wounded in the hospital: "how sternly they contrasted with the man who had attempted suicide! Yet did they contrast, after all? Were they finer, nobler, than he?"[41] she wonders. While searching for the difference between the men, she concludes that "the difference lay in the Ideal. One had no ideals. The others had ideals, and fought for them."[42] Even this important distinction between the suicidal soldier and his peers is negated when she reviews the other men's characters and behavior: "poor selfish Alexandre, poor vain Félix, poor gluttonous Alphonse, poor filthy Hippolyte–was it possible that each cherished ideals, hidden beneath? Courageous dreams of freedom and patriotism?"[43] She determines that men have no innate ideals, but rather are "base metal, gilded."[44] The gilding comes from "somewhere, higher up, a handful of men had been able to impose … a state of mind" on these soldiers.[45] Ideals do not emerge from the men themselves, who only need to provide their bodies and put them at the service of the state. She writes, "individual nobility was superfluous. All the Idealists demanded was physical endurance from the mass."[46] This story puts forth a strong critique of the military and the hospital system that strips the "mass" of men in its ranks of will and distinctiveness, leading the narrator to question the meaningfulness of work, both soldiering and nursing, typically invested with nobility.[47]

The editors of the *Atlantic Monthly* felt compelled to defend their decision to publish this controversial piece. In the following month's issue, they explained that:

> The savage little sketch … was not published to be popular. We printed it with all its apparent bitterness and cruelty because it served, as only the truth can, to show the artificial standards which war creates. The virtues which war extols are not the normal virtues; a soldier's faults may be a citizen's salvation. People are too apt, under stress of the well-nigh unbearable strain of the war, to believe that after this martyrdom there will be a resurrection of nations glorified and made perfect.[48]

Two letters subsequently published in the November 1916 issue demonstrate why the editors may have felt compelled to explain the reason they published such a bluntly written piece. The writers of the letters challenge La Motte's depiction of the selfish and self-destructive behaviors of the French soldiers, offering a counterargument to her vision with their own firsthand experiences of hospitals in wartime France as being full of soldiers they praise for "their patience, their gratitude, their self-control under intense pain, and their deep appreciation of everything that is done for them."[49] The reason for defending the French character becomes evident later in the same letter when the writer implores the American public:

> Dear American people, you who are citizens of a great Sister Republic, you who have lived and fought for ideals, you who are now showing the world so noble an example of generosity, not only in the ceaseless stream of supplies of all kinds that you are pouring into this stricken land, but in the giving cheerfully, endlessly, the service–yes, and the *lives* of your dear ones, do not believe that they for whom you are making such sacrifices are unworthy of them. They are deserving of all of your great gifts: they receive them with deepest thankfulness, with deepest appreciation.[50]

The primary concern is that La Motte's "Heroes" would stem the tide of generous donations making their way to hospitals like the American Ambulances in Juilly and Neuilly by betraying the image of the wounded soldier as long-suffering and docile. This criticism had also been lodged against La Motte in the wake of her publication of "An American Nurse in Paris" in the *Survey* in July 1915. In response to that piece critiquing the wastefulness of the American Ambulance in Neuilly,[51] Frank H. Mason, identified as Chairman of American Ambulance Committee, wrote a rebuttal to her depiction of the hospital by drawing on a report written by "Dr. J. William White, professor emeritus of surgery at the University of Pennsylvania, … an experienced and recognized authority in every detail of hospital management."[52] White's observations of the hospital, made in July 1915, were that "it has been run most intelligently and with that sense of a proper proportion between necessary and unnecessary economies, and of the difference between extravagance and wise liberality, which marks capable hospital management."[53] La Motte, briefly described as "a trained nurse who served in the American Ambulance Hospital at Neuilly for a period of about three weeks in November, 1914,"[54] and her perspective are intended to be soundly refuted by White's superior expertise and firsthand experience.

If readers who did not know La Motte were insulted and outraged by her representation of hospitals and patients in her articles, those who did know her and worked alongside her were even more upset by her writings, particularly after the publication of *The Backwash of War* in the fall of 1916. Presumably her success publishing in the *Atlantic Monthly* gave her hope that she could find a wider audience for her writings that explored her nursing expertise and experiences in fictional sketches. The experiments in fiction that she had been working on in Paris before the war,[55] though never published, had helped to prepare her for writing in this new form, and by June 1916 Mary E. Lent, acting as La Motte's go-between once again, sent the sketches to Putnam's. The initial reaction to them was not positive. Though La Motte was lightly praised for her ability "to observe and … describe" the editor felt that the sketches were best suited to "periodical publication" and turned down the collection for fear it would not generate enough income in a market "saturated with material about the war, and with personal experiences, whether of the soilders [*sic*] or of non-combatants."[56]

Notwithstanding this rejection, a month later, a letter from George H. Putnam himself, then president of the publishing firm, offered her a contract, stipulating that she add an introduction in which she "will give an account of the author's experience at the front, and will make clear the special purpose she has in mind for writing this book."[57] His desire for the introduction stemmed from his, and other readers' from Putnam's, lack of clarity regarding the goal of the collection. Putnam explained that:

> It is my individual opinion that the truthfulness of the pictures would have been better emphasized with the general reader (I have myself no question as to the absolute accuracy of the statement) if the author had not restricted her episodes to these scenes of misery and horror. The picture would, as a whole, have been more trustworthy and more valuable. Some of my associates are, however, of the impression that your volume has been prepared as a peace tract and that you had perhaps thought best to restrict your selections to the scenes of misery.[58]

The misunderstanding that she was an ardent pacifist promoted the book with readers sympathetic to pacifism, such as the staff and readers of socialist publications like the *Masses*. Max Eastman, editor of the *Masses* and co-founder with his sister, Crystal Eastman, of its successor, the *Liberator*,[59] explained that La Motte was named as contributing editor to the *Liberator*–her name appeared on the masthead from March through October 1918–though she was "merely a name on our masthead placed there because she had written *The Backwash of War*, a little book we all admired … She was a passerby."[60] The *Masses* communicated its strong support for the book in the January 1917 volume in which W. G. Fuller, a British editor married to Crystal Eastman, reviewed it, ironically invoking Florence Nightingale in the title of his review, "The Lady of the Lamp," exclaiming that "it is a bitter, angry laugh at Churches, at discipline, nationalism, patriotism, at the whole military system, at the crime and madness of War."[61] Floyd Dell, the managing editor, added a paragraph after Fuller's review to explain:

> I cannot refrain from adding my praise to his admirable account of that book. It is, it seems to me, a book more likely than any other so far produced by the war, to last beyond the war. And this, not because it describes war's horrors, but because it describes them with a curious anæsthesia. It tells unsparingly all that there is to tell–all that has never been told before–but with a quality of art which partly anæsthetizes some of the emotions and appeals directly to the mind–a tremendous artistic achievement. If you don't want to miss one of the best books written in the last ten years in the English language, you must read this book.[62]

This praise from one of Greenwich Village's leading leftist thinkers must have been flattering for La Motte, who had been striving for years to move beyond writing professionally about nursing and to earn an audience for her creative writing. The recognition of her book by the *Masses* may also have put her in contact with Heterodoxy, a loosely organized club for radical women that met from 1912 to 1940 in Greenwich Village, of which Crystal Eastman was also a member. Many prominent suffrage activists, such as Mary Ware Dennett, Alison Turnbull Hopkins, and Marie Jenney Howe, were also members of the group and La Motte could also have been encouraged to attend meetings through the suffrage network.[63]

While receiving the validation of the bohemians of Greenwich was undoubtedly satisfying, given La Motte's family's conservative political views coupled with the scrutiny the *Masses* faced when the government brought charges against it in 1917, her brief association with the magazine was undoubtedly unwanted. At any rate, Eastman's reading of the pacifist intent was erroneous, if understandable. La Motte never professed any belief in an idealistic view of the power of literature to combat war, and she did not see the line between peace and war as being as well defined as pacifists did. In fact, in her diary she recorded one conversation with two French nurses in which they discussed "a dying man, & they shrugged their shoulders 'c'est la guerre.' So it is–some how I cannot think or feel that this awful tragedy of death is worse than the awful tragedy of life."[64] Putnam too could only view her stark and bitter stories through the pacifist lens and concluded, "We have arrived at the opinion that notwithstanding the sombreness of your series of sketches, the volume, as you have planned it, ought to come into print and will be likely to attract a satisfactory measure of attention."[65] The volume was subsequently in circulation by the fall of 1916 and elicited strong reactions from those with whom La Motte had served in France.

Agnes Warner was an experienced nurse who joined the hospital on September 24, 1915 and was one of the rare recipients of La Motte's approval. After their initial meeting, La Motte briefly observed, "Miss Warner came tonight, from Paris. First impression very favorable."[66] Warner, loyal to Borden Turner, ended up staying with her for the duration of the war and believed in their nursing mission and the nobility of the French soldier. Her perspective on the war was expressed through a compilation of her letters assembled by her friends to raise money for the hospital and published without her knowledge as *My Beloved Poilus* in March 1917. The title accurately communicates her warm affection and deep respect for her patients. Given Warner's devotion to them and the hospital, it is unsurprising that she reacted negatively to the publication of *The Backwash of War*. In a letter to Maud Mortimer Clapp, sent before Warner knew that her collection of letters would soon be published, Warner asked, "By the way, have you read Miss La Motte's book? I have not seen it yet, but all those who have are most indignant about it. They say it gives one such a terrible idea of the French–of the hospital. You have been here and you know what wonderful men they were & how courageous & you know what the whole tone of the hospital was. Couldn't you write something to counteract the impression her book has made?"[67]

Without having actually read the book at this point, Warner was sufficiently concerned about the damage La Motte was doing to the reputation of the hospital to seek out someone who could potentially write a countertext to the grim vision of nursing and soldiering in La Motte's slim volume. Warner, and presumably Borden Turner, must have been particularly horrified by the dedication to "Mary Borden-Turner, 'The Little Boss,' to whom I owe my experience in the zone of the armies," which appeared in the first printing. La Motte came to see the error of dedicating a volume shot through with critiques of the war, the hospital system, and the men who served to someone still serving as the *directrice* of a frontline military hospital. She wrote to Putnam's in July 1917, soliciting a reply that the publisher would omit the dedication from subsequent printings.[68] The letter also refers obliquely to consternation on the part of the French government and the publisher's response: "We wrote to the French government in reply to their kick and politely told them to go to. I do not believe you will have any difficulty if you go back there."[69] Clearly, both the government and individuals still fighting the war found much to which they objected in the text.[70]

If the French authorities were unhappy with La Motte's representations of hospital life, her acquaintances from the hospital were more so. Clapp, whose response to Warner does not survive, was happy to comply with her request that she produce a countertext to *The Backwash of War*. Motivated by her extreme dislike of La Motte and by a desire to articulate her personal experiences, she eventually published *A Green Tent in Flanders*. Her first foray into sharing her hospital experiences came in the October 1916 issue of the *Atlantic Monthly*, in which she shared publication space with La Motte. Based on the hostile views she held of La Motte by then, Clapp undoubtedly resented this coincidence immensely. She did not always feel so negatively about La Motte, however. In a letter from 1913, Clapp refers to La Motte with regard to her help with a family matter, explaining, "We owe her a great deal of gratitude for giving us Miss La Motte. I have lost my heart to her & Tim won't admit how much he likes her which is always a bad sign!"[71] While what La Motte did for Clapp is not specified in the letter, Clapp's warmth and enthusiasm for her is evident.

Their relationship would remain cordial for at least the following two years. In May 1915, La Motte procured glasses for Clapp and sent them to her in London, along with an excited description of her recent conversation with Borden Turner and her decision to take La Motte on; the letter is evidence that Clapp first heard of Borden Turner and the hospital through La Motte and the news inspired Clapp with a mix of feelings. She wrote to her husband a few days later, referring to La Motte's news as "wonderful for her," but that she was "filled with envy!"[72] She was also prompted to write to ask if the hospital could use her husband as "orderly, or translator or something, & me as ??"[73] She followed this declaration with the wistful observation, "*Mon Dieu* how I have wasted my life that I can go as nothing but housemaid, I who was so vain."[74]

La Motte maintained her correspondence with Clapp after beginning her employment with Borden Turner, explaining several months later that she knew of no job for her, but that she would "look sharp" on her behalf.[75] True to her word, the next month, La Motte wrote to Clapp in response to a letter that has not survived, but in which Clapp must have persisted in her inquiries regarding the possibility of obtaining a position, to explain "I don't believe there is a bit of chance of getting you here. There is just one such position, occupied by a layman–just such as you would like & enjoy & could do admirably–but it is filled by an English woman, a friend of Mrs. Turner's. She spoke lately of giving it up & going back to England, & I was waiting to put in my word for you when she changed her mind & decided to stay."[76] La Motte continued with her explanation, making a point that would later become a source of profound irritation for Clapp: "The rest of us are all fully trained nurses, & as there are only a few of us, Mrs. T. wants to keep the staff of such entirely."[77] The message to Mortimer had to be clear: untrained women, used in significant numbers in other hospitals during the war, were not wanted or needed in Borden Turner's.

As Clapp's comment to her husband about being unskilled to do anything but work as a "housemaid" revealed, she was insecure and frustrated at her inability to make a meaningful contribution to the war effort. Born in 1875, Clapp was the daughter of English parents, her father, Edward Ede, a lawyer working for the Metropolitan Life Insurance Company of New York.[78] She was educated at various art schools in Europe and married Frederick Mortimer Clapp, who became the first director of the Frick Collection in 1936, in 1908.[79]

The two did not have any surviving children, though in 1912 Clapp gave birth to a stillborn daughter in Switzerland. This event was undoubtedly devastating for the couple, however little Clapp said about it in surviving letters, such as in the middle of a newsy letter written in August 1912, when she told her mother-in-law that "we can in no way reconcile ourselves to our loss; we see so many nice babies everywhere & can never for a moment forget our charming little girl."[80] These few lines are the extent of the grief she permitted herself to share before returning to her discussion of family news and their plans to leave Switzerland and return to Italy. By this time Clapp was in her early forties and either through choice or necessity, the couple did not have any other children. When the war broke out, she did not have children to occupy her attention and she was searching for a way to feel useful and needed, a common enough sentiment among the women of her class who had never embarked on careers that would have prepared them to contribute in an obvious way to the war effort.

Her wish to find a position later came to fruition in November 1915 when La Motte wrote to her in Italy to tell her that Mrs. Abraham, the woman who had been filling the job La Motte believed would suit Clapp perfectly, had left the hospital. She took time to describe the job as "consist[ing] in taking charge of the linen room and surgical supplies, portioning them out on demand, etc., and also in receiving the patients in the *Salle d'Attente*, just as they are brought in from the ambulances, where they are cleaned up before being sent to the wards."[81] One part of the job, as La Motte presents it, does not require any nursing expertise but only organizational skills and the capacity for monotonous work. The business of receiving patients sounds like nursing work according to today's standards, but apparently La Motte viewed it as a task any "layman" could perform successfully, though she would, to Clapp's intense aggravation, later revise her opinion and campaign to have trained nurses in the receiving ward.

La Motte was finished with the war–or so she asserted in her letter at the time, informing Clapp that "Unfortunately, I am not there any longer, as I got enough of it, and perhaps after all my being there was part of the inducement."[82] She continued to entice Clapp to accept the position by describing the relative comfort of the hospital and the qualities of Borden Turner, "a dandy" La Motte felt Clapp would like.[83] Clapp must have written right back to express her interest; a letter from La Motte to Clapp, written less than two weeks after her original letter, tells Clapp that she has written to Borden Turner to communicate her interest and that she should expect direct communication from her if the position were to open up. It did so soon thereafter, since Clapp wrote to her husband at the end of November that she had received a telegram from Borden Turner and was ready to embark for the hospital, taking La Motte up on her offer to stay in her apartment at 21, rue Vaneau in the seventh *arrondissement* as she passed through Paris on her way to the hospital. Later, in *A Green Tent in Flanders*, Clapp described La Motte's apartment–though without identifying it–providing a rare glimpse into La Motte's personal space, "kindly lent" to Clapp. La Motte had decorated this "pretty little perch" with "war trophies," including "empty shell cases and hand grenades" and "lumps of shrapnel" and proclamations issued by German authorities to the people of Liège and Charleroi,[84] "trophies" La Motte described buying in her diary in mid-June before her departure for Dunkirk.[85]

Clapp's time in Paris was plagued with difficulties getting her paperwork in order despite having a letter from Borden Turner proving she needed to travel to the war zone. While still in Paris, she settled her financial affairs and described socializing with Chadbourne, who invited her to lunch and a concert, and La Motte. La Motte shared some writing with her, presumably a draft copy of "Heroes," which Clapp described as "brutal, vivid, and good."[86] Clapp's journey to the hospital, however, would be less prolonged than La Motte's much-thwarted attempt to get to the front during the first half of 1915, and by December 16 she was in Dunkirk.

She arrived at the hospital that La Motte had left almost two months earlier, a place that La Motte found trying because of the discord amongst the medical staff and the senselessness of nursing those destined to be killed on the front lines. She had warned Clapp about the "jealousies & quarrels" in the hospital, and Clapp believed that her "billet would not touch them."[87] La Motte had also tired of feeling as if her skills were being wasted. In one of her last diary entries about nursing in Belgium, she observed:

> [J]ust as I am getting ready to leave, 2 sick men arrive. Miss Warner can manage, however. Am very tired, & feel I can do so little here–so little in comparison to my possibilities & training, that I am just wasting myself.

> Rouhier, for all he likes me, won't trust me to give a dose of medicine. Gives all his orders to the Sergeant, & permits the pts. to have a bottle of chloral hydrate back of his bed, & to help himself.[88]

Presumably, Clapp's lack of nursing responsibilities was to shield her from these conflicts among nurses coming from different nursing backgrounds and practices. Since she had no nursing skills, she did not fear that her talents would be wasted.

However, Clapp's letters make clear that she envied the nurses and their sense of purpose in the hospital. Her position as the overseer of the supply room was plainly not nursing work, but her position in the *salle d'attente*, where she received and washed the wounded, brought her into contact with the men and encouraged a greater interest in nursing duties. She described to her husband, "I get so attached to these men & wish in a way, I had the training to have a ward–on the other hand although I do not come so near them, I see most of the [game]."[89] She was allowed to satisfy her desire to see more of the patients she received in the *salle d'attente* by "pay[ing] them extra little visits" in the wards and shadowing Warner, who encouraged Clapp's interest in learning more about nursing procedures.[90]

Clapp's attempts to watch and learn more about nursing practices would be thwarted by the return of La Motte to the hospital on January 17, 1916.[91] There would develop between the two of them the kind of "well-documented conflict between trained nurses and volunteers in hospitals" that occurred in many wartime hospitals.[92] La Motte had been absent for a period of three months, during which she traveled in Spain with Chadbourne and spent time in Paris where she worked on "Heroes" and "La Patrie Reconnaissante" in December 1915, shortly after Clapp left her apartment for the hospital. While La Motte had asserted to Clapp in the fall of 1915 that she was done with war nursing, she returned for a temporary work stint at the behest of Borden Turner. Clapp had been friendly with La Motte up until this point and had expressed little ambivalence about her return in her letters to her husband–her only question being whether she would still be needed once La Motte returned–yet their relationship took a different turn once put under the pressure of the working conditions in the hospital and their subsequent clashing over their divergent understandings of what kind of nursing belonged in the hospital.

Within two days, Clapp started writing letters to her husband in which she complained that La Motte had put her things in Borden Turner's room, to be "in command," and that "perhaps I ought to feel offended but don't–after all she has been here for 3 months before & is an organizer & hates not to be cock of the walk."[93] Clapp's protestations that she was not offended soon ceased and her hostility toward La Motte increased as La Motte's presence in the hospital changed the dynamics, at least from Clapp's point of view, of the functioning of the wards. Clapp chafed when she wanted access to La Motte's ward to visit "a friend of mine who was dying,"[94] but La Motte told her "you had better go away now."[95] La Motte later made clear that "it is not professional to have people in the ward."[96] Apparently, La Motte's behavior fell outside of what other nurses found permissible, as Clapp explained: "All the other nurses are dear & nice to me but they do not compare for training & knowledge to Warner or Ellen."[97] In the case of La Motte, despite feeling resentful at the way she treated her, Clapp had to give her grudging respect because of her great nursing skill, but that skill combined with La Motte's strongly expressed views of her professional nursing expectations combined to create tension in their relationship, at least from the perspective of Clapp. A clash between the French and the Americans during which Clapp "took the French side, she the American" augmented the difficulties between them.[98] Even as Clapp wrote to her husband to express her bitterness, in the same letter she tried to reassure him, "Don't think E. & I have strained relations."[99] This prevarication is typical of her letters, in which Clapp fears being perceived as petty and tries to undo her own words that communicate the escalating tensions in the hospital and her insecurities about finding a place in it when she had no trained nursing skills.

Clapp's resentments grew more profound with La Motte, calling her "executive & red tape," language she would invoke in her caricature of La Motte in *A Green Tent in Flanders*, for wanting "to put one of the 'nurses' in the Salle d'Attente" because "It is a nurse's job."[100] The threat of losing this contact with the men led her to muse that "If they take that away from me I doubt whether I stay."[101] The distance between the approaches to care held by the two women, one highly trained, the other with no nursing skills, became more evident when La Motte told Clapp that she was "a mush of sentimentality," causing Clapp to write angrily to her husband that La Motte was "like a knife for organization."[102] In the same letter, Clapp expressed her sense of betrayal at La Motte's forcing her out of nursing opportunities and reflected that "Humanity, no women, are beasts. I used to think I liked them. I really despise them–but this is just spleen, take it for what it is worth."[103] Her vitriol about women stands in sharp contrast to the men she describes in the next sentence as "wonderful, patient, thoughtful, brave."[104] With regard to them, Clapp gives them the deference and respect to which she presumably believed men were entitled, magnified by their sacrifice and suffering during the war. However, her deep ambivalence about being in an environment in which women wielded power and influence and worked with great professionalism is evident when, after explaining to her husband that her inability to navigate the intrigues of the hospital was due to her having "been really too little with human beings except with isolated specimens," she then says with relief that she is "glad to have a prospect of being out of the world before the women are in power."[105]

Clapp's uneasiness with inhabiting a world shaped by women was exacerbated by her discomfiture with what she perceived as the class differences at work, creating a fraught atmosphere between her, Borden Turner, and La Motte. She described La Motte as being "hand in glove with all these wealthy people. I am something they use & who uses them."[106] Clapp's rather odd assessment that as a volunteer in a war hospital she was being taken advantage of illustrates her ambivalent attitude toward the worth of her work and her place in relation to her social betters. She complained to her husband on several occasions about feeling "isolated" as a result of her status in the hospital. She described herself as "neither a nurse–& I seem to perceive that perhaps it is a sort of professional jealousy against the despised V.A.D which I so humbly represent–nor a directress, nor a housekeeper, yet expected to be all."[107] While most VADs were from wealthy families,[108] Clapp could not, in relation to Borden Turner and La Motte, compensate for her inferior position in the hospital with a sense of class and social superiority. Rather, she had neither the authority and money of Borden Turner nor the nursing skill of La Motte, all of which left her completing work she described as "stupid, keeping up the fires making toast & tea, writing letters."[109] This necessary labor appeared frivolous in her eyes, and, combined with "all this nurses etiquette," kept her from "real touch with the *blessés* outside my own *Salle d'Attente*."[110] Her ego bruised and the distance from her husband pressing on her, she declared "I prepare to make my *malles* & depart very soon," and left the hospital on March 16 for Paris, where she stayed until she made her way back to the United States in April 1916.

The experience left Clapp with intense bitterness toward La Motte, something she would excise to a degree by writing *A Green Tent in Flanders*, getting her revenge by caricaturing La Motte's penchant for order and inflexibility. Clapp guarded the anonymity of the people about whom she wrote in the text, a mechanism that allowed her to split her representation of La Motte without the reader being aware that she was presenting the same person as though she were several different people. For example, Clapp describes La Motte's apartment, an account that matches those in her letters to her husband and in her diary, where she clearly states that she is staying in La Motte's home, but never comments on any of the attributes of her host; she only introduces La Motte directly when she discusses leaving for the train station in preparation for going to the front and being joined by "a friend" who "is just back from the front and from the hopelessness of patching people up only to be killed or further mutilated when they don't want to be either."[111] Additionally, the "friend" tells Clapp, "Heroism in war is nothing but a reflection from above–imitation or coercion–not skin deep and therefore of no value to the individual,"[112] echoing themes explored in *The Backwash of War*.

Later in *A Green Tent in Flanders*, Clapp does not connect this "friend" embittered by war nursing to the woman she witheringly calls "Organization" and to whom she devotes a brief chapter.[113] Though "Organization" "has the pleasantest ways and a witty good fellowship" she "adores uniformity" and is "almost cubistic in her dire simplifications."[114] Clapp builds a more damning portrait by claiming that she "has done with nursing" despite being "a fully trained and excellent nurse" and is not at the hospital "to probe physical weakness but to cut deeper–for the purification of art and sentiment–down to the unquestionable depravity of the human heart."[115] Having accumulated the experiences required, "Organization" leaves with her "attaché case bulg[ing] with documentary evidence of the obliquity of human nature especially as observed under torture in a field hospital."[116]

While La Motte apparently left the hospital in the latter part of February 1916 with some kind of record of her time there, those papers or diary have not survived. What is left behind to contest Clapp's one-dimensional depiction of her is *The Backwash of War*, published a year before Clapp's book. To be fair, Clapp's observation that La Motte was no longer interested in nursing was an apt one. She had burned out on her chosen profession in 1913 when she took her leave from the Baltimore Health Department, and though the war offered a kind of intense nursing experience that was new to her, in the end, the routines of the wards were the same as those in peacetime and she found no nobility of purpose in taking part in the machinery of war. As one of her narrators observes, "This is war. But it goes on and on … till it seems like life. Life in peace time. It might be life in a big city hospital, so alike is the routine."[117] For her, war brought out the extremes of experience or characteristics in people and laid bare all that is "weak, hideous, [and] repellent."[118] She refused to idealize the men who fought the war and those who cared for them; instead, she wrote unrelentingly about human suffering and degradation. She also laid bare the hypocrisies at work in the rhetoric of war commonly employed to present soldiers as saints and medical professionals as martyrs, and she contested those depictions by portraying them as normal human beings with foibles the same as those they possessed in peacetime. As she so often did, La Motte took events from her experiences and used them as the basis for her writing and as a mechanism for exploring the shortcomings of those around her. For example, according to Clapp's diary, La Motte told her that "the old médecin chef had a cult for young girls used to go into Rousbrugge every night 'respectable girls' as no others are allowed about here."[119] If it was an "open secret" that the doctor made these visits, undoubtedly few associated with the hospital would appreciate La Motte sharing it with the general public, yet she used the incident as the kernel for a story that explores the hypocritical sexual behavior of men.

Having represented soldiers in "Heroes" as selfish and vain, rejecting the tendency to idealize them, in "Women and Wives" La Motte attacks the hypocrisy of the male medical staff in their relationships with women. The narrator, a nurse in *Salle I*, tells the reader, "War, superb as it is, is not necessarily a filtering process, by which men and nations may be purified. Well, there are many people to write you of the noble side, the heroic side, the exalted side of war. I must write you of what I have seen, the other side, the backwash. They are both true."[120] La Motte uses the rainy, cold winter setting to advantage, thus creating an environment so dreary and unappealing that the reader anticipates no "superb" action is forthcoming. Rather, the story develops prosaically, with the bored patients in *Salle I* showing the nurse photographs of their wives and children. She remarks that they were "pathetic little pictures … of common, working-class women, some fat and work-worn, some thin and work-worn."[121] Her condescending tone continues as she assesses the significance of these women, "the stupid, ordinary wives [who] represented home. And the words home and wife were interchangeable and stood for the same thing."[122] Yet, as the story progresses, it becomes evident that the source of her anger and derision is not the wives themselves, but the men who idealize and then betray them.

The medical staff in the hospital share the soldiers' understanding of women and home; the nurse reveals that Armand, "the chief orderly," and Simon, "the young surgeon," too have wives about whom they share stories and from whom they anxiously await letters.[123] The nurse, however, begins to take apart this depiction of dedicated husbands as she describes how wives are not allowed to visit their husbands in the "War Zone" because they "are bad for the morale of the Army. They come with their troubles, to talk of how business is failing, of how things are going to the bad at home."[124] Women, however, are allowed in "because they cheer and refresh the troops."[125] Armand and Simon take advantage of these morale-boosting women–both go into the village to visit a girl on a regular basis, which prompts the narrator to ask angrily, "why does [Simon] talk so incessantly about his wife, and show her pictures to me, to every one about the place? Why should we all be bored with tales of Simon's stupid wife, when that's all she means to him?"[126] Even one of the doctors, aged sixty-four, "goes down to our village for a little girl of fourteen. He was decorated with the Legion of Honour the other day. It seems incongruous."[127]

La Motte's long history as an advocate for women's suffrage and her work as a court reporter for the *New Voter*, during which she exposed the hypocrisies of the judicial system in relation to the treatment of women, prepared her to lay bare the iniquities between men and women.[128] In the power dynamic depicted in the story, men yearn for the security and familiarity represented by their wives, symbols of the comforts of home, but need not extend any loyalty to them. These same men are praised for their loyalty to their nations during the war and any betrayal of it would be met with a court martial, but there is no censure of them for betraying their wives to meet their sexual needs. They are not judged, either, for the effects of their behavior on the local female population. The narrator sarcastically comments, "it's not the men's fault that most of the women in the War Zone are ruined … the professional prostitutes from Paris aren't admitted to the War Zone, but the Belgian girls made such fools of themselves, the others weren't needed."[129] In contrast to the way the Belgian women throw themselves at French men, they are coerced by the Germans, according to Allied propaganda, because "it is inconceivable how any decent girl, even a Belgian, could give herself up voluntarily to a Hun! They used force, those brutes!"[130] The power of the story comes from its unrelenting revelations of the hypocrisy of those men, hailed as heroes for their healing prowess, who take advantage of vulnerable women in the War Zone while holding up their wives as beloved symbols of the virtues of home.

While rejecting the rhetoric of heroism, whether as applied to soldiers or those caring for them, La Motte nonetheless expresses profound sorrow for the damaging effects of the war on those caught in the crossfire, the men whose bodies bore the brunt of its violence, and the minds of those caring for them. Her articulation of this suffering emerges from a focus on the waste produced by the destructiveness of the war. She initiated this theme in her first piece about war nursing, "An American Nurse in Paris," in which she describes the economic waste generated by the American Hospital.[131] Her later writings give voice to the enormous waste of human life she witnessed in the frontline hospital. In "Heroes" she forces the reader to engage with how human life is assessed and valued in the hospital environment, where resources, such as the surgeon's time and medical supplies, are available in limited quantities. She returns to this preoccupation in "A Belgian Civilian," another story fleshed out using La Motte's personal experiences. However, the diary treats the incident with more compassion than the fictive version does. La Motte recorded briefly in two lines, "A small Belgian boy was just now brought in (10 p.m.) having been hit in the abdomen by a piece of shell, at Ypres. Too weak to stand an [anesthetic]. Dr. Rouget greatly upset."[132] She updated this brief sketch the next day with a more prolonged discussion, noting:

> The little Belgian boy op. on this a.m. Multiple perforations of the intestines & general [?]. The Englishmen who brought him in last night brought his mother this afternoon. At first she seemed apathetic & indifferent–more from shock & the [?] events of the past months however. The shell burst in their kitchen, & injured another child as well. Her husband keeps an inn at a village outside of Ypres–she has been urging him to refuge in England, but he has been postponing it, unwilling to give up his little home & livelihood. The child died tonight at 11:30 p.m. Our first death.[133]

According to this account the surgeon and the mother feel distress at the sight of this terribly injured boy; however, La Motte transmutes their concerns into indifference and annoyance in her fictional depiction of the event and has her narrator describe how an exceptional case was brought in by an English ambulance, an unusual event in the French military hospital, but the medical staff realize it is "only a small Belgian boy, a civilian, and Belgian civilians belong neither to the French nor the English services."[134] Yet, he is "dump[ed] … at this French hospital … to get rid of him the sooner. In war, civilians are cheap things at best, and an immature civilian, Belgian at that, is very cheap."[135] The dilemma of having to care for a body that has no worth to the larger cause of the war is magnified when it is clear that "it was a hopeless case, anyhow. The child would die without an operation, or he would die during the operation, or he would die after the operation."[136] Faced with wasting his time and the hospital's resources, the surgeon grudgingly performs the operation, and afterwards the child is a disruptive presence on the ward: "Being ten years of age, he was unreasonable, and bawled for [his mother] incessantly and could not be pacified. The patients were greatly annoyed … and there was indignation that the welfare and comfort of useful soldiers should be interfered with by the whims of a futile and useless civilian."[137] The child's life cannot be redeemed even by maternal love: the *Directrice* summons the boy's mother, believing "a mother's place was with her child, if that child was dying," but the mother, busy taking care of her bar in a nearby city, rails against being "dragged away from her home, from her family" to attend her son's dying.[138] The end result is that the child dies uncared for and is buried perfunctorily after his mother has left to return to her family and business, underlining the mercantile quality of exchanges between individuals in the hospital. The boy has no value to the French, the military, the patients and staff in the hospital, or even to his own mother, whose love, though expressed, is overcome by her desire to continue making money "selling drink to the English soldiers."[139]

Other kinds of unvalued citizens are examined in "A Citation," in which Grammont, sent to serve in the *Bataillons d'Afrique* instead of going to prison for being a thief (the *bataillons* were typically made up of men with criminal records or soldiers with a bad service record), comes to the hospital having been shot in the spleen. In "A Belgian Civilian" and "Heroes" the narrator interrogates the uselessness of wasting expensive resources on those who cannot be saved or who serve no larger purpose in the war; in this story, the narrator critiques the extending of care, observing that "had [Grammont] died promptly, as he should have done, it would have been better."[140] Dying quickly would have spared Grammont the attention of "a surgeon connected with the hospital who was bent on making a reputation for himself, and this consisted in trying to prolong the lives of wounded men who ought normally and naturally to have died."[141] It is undoubtedly in part Grammont's status as a criminal that emboldens the doctor to experiment on him with expensive techniques; the narrator notes that Grammont endures the painful operations quietly and "did not ask to be allowed to die, as many of them did, for since he was of the *Bataillon d'Afrique*, such a request would be equivalent to asking for a remission of sentence."[142] Rather, he tolerates the efforts of the surgeon, who "worked hand in hand with the *Directrice* who wanted her hospital to make a reputation for saving the lives of the *grands blessés*."[143]

During his travail, the nurse notices Grammont's capacity for quiet endurance as he undergoes life-prolonging treatments for five months. She comes to recognize that he has "rather heroic qualities of endurance, of bravery, of discipline … developed by months of extreme agony, of extreme bodily pain."[144] The *Directrice* consequently exercises her influence to pressure the General to award Grammont a citation, having discovered that he possessed the same capacity for heroic behavior in battle. The award, never given to the criminals of the *Bataillon d'Afrique*, after much delay is finally going to be awarded, and "it was a condescension that he should be so honored at all."[145] As with all of her stories, this one ends on a cruel and ironic note: Grammont dies "twenty minutes before the General arrived with his medals."[146] The reader is left to ponder the purpose of Grammont's prolonged suffering and the inhumanity of the hospital system that used him to further its own ends without considering the cost to the patient. For the narrator, these efforts are wasted, not because Grammont does not merit the care–her admiration and concern for him is evident throughout the story and motivates her criticism of the surgeon and *Directrice*–but because they serve the ego and selfish motivations of others instead of the patient. She further hammers home institutional indifference to the individuals who serve the war effort, particularly those at the bottom of the social hierarchy, like the *joyeux*, Grammont, when the General arrives too late to award the citation even though the other men in the ward received theirs in a much shorter period of time. The story highlights the waste and futility of what is construed as "care" in the military hospital and the way that patients are vulnerable to being made to serve the goals of others.

Of course, the same accusation could be lodged against La Motte and was by Clapp, though she too would transform her experiences in the hospital into book form. As Clapp claimed, La Motte had tired of nursing, yet she went to the hospital anyway, and as her diary makes clear, while she found the waste of life that she heard about because of the poor medical conditions of French hospitals terrible and felt she had important skills as a trained nurse that could alleviate suffering, she also wanted, like many men and women who volunteered to serve, to be part of the experience and, presumably, to write about it. The diary does not express any guilt over that wish; however, several of her stories reveal ambivalence about using the suffering of others to serve personal ends. She indicts the surgeon and *Directrice* in "A Citation" and hints at her own complicity in several pieces in the collection. In "La Patrie Reconnaissante" an angry patient, Marius, is brought to the hospital. While cursing the stretcher-bearers for taking so long to get to him, he fixes his attention on "Americans in khaki, ruddy, well fed, careless."[147] In his estimation, for these healthy Americans, the war is an adventure for which they have volunteered to perform safe jobs. Their reasons for doing so are not revealed, but Marius offers an interpretation of their motivations for being in France in 1915: "What are they here for–France? No, only themselves! To write a book–to say what they have done–when it was safe!"[148] The Americans are questioned for mining the war for material for artistic productions, and La Motte's own body of writing appears indirectly subject to this same critique. Her defense, however, is the content of the stories themselves. In her capacity as an artist she expands the role of witness that she takes on as a nurse. When she cannot cure, alleviate pain, or attest to a man's death, she can write his pain, translating the suffering of the dying body into print.

One of the most powerful stories in *The Backwash of War*, "Alone," does this work and serves as a testament to the death of one soldier. In the story, written in April 1916 after La Motte's second trip to the hospital, the narrator describes a dying man, Rochard, who is the subject of intense interest on the part of the doctors in training at the field hospital. Yet, all the available medical technology can neither heal the serious wound, now gangrenous, to Rochard's thigh nor alleviate his excruciating pain. As Rochard sinks into a senseless state, the narrator reflects, "No one ...was fond of Rochard. He had only been there a few hours. He meant nothing to any one there. He was a dying man, in a field hospital, that was all."[149] For his life and death to have meaning there must be a witness present to record the moment and save this particular *poilu* from oblivion. The nurses who care for him have the potential to serve in that capacity; the narrator comments that "the nurse cared for him very gently, very conscientiously, very skillfully."[150] Yet, this "care" is of an abstract, remote kind administered with emotional disengagement. In the end, "Rochard died, a stranger among strangers. And there were many people there to wait upon him, but there was no one there to love him."[151] The nurse can provide him with solicitous attention, yet she cannot grant the love that would preserve this man from a lonely death.

Nevertheless, the nurse's concern for Rochard belies her insistence on her strictly professional interest in her patient. She must leave him to go to lunch, but instructs the orderly to warn her if there is any change in her charge. She returns "and hurried to see Rochard, hurried behind the flamboyant, red, cheerful screens that shut him off from the rest of the ward. Rochard was dead."[152] Her anxiety for Rochard is evident in her rush to return to him, yet her efforts are useless. The nurse's earlier mocking of medical technology is echoed in these final lines. The hospital and staff have failed Rochard in every way: they could not treat him, alleviate his suffering, or even testify to the moment of his death.

The narrator compensates for the nurse's absence and consequent inability to witness Rochard's death by writing the story "Alone," ensuring that the circumstances surrounding his lonely death are recorded, thereby redeeming his anonymity in the hospital. The narrator of "At the Telephone" takes on a similar role. She watches a man with a mortal wound being operated on to give him a "one in a thousand" or maybe only a "one in ten thousand" chance to survive.[153] He babbles as he undergoes the operation in too precarious a position to be given a general anesthetic. As his condition worsens during the grueling operation, "his remarks grew less coherent, and he seemed to find himself back in the trenches, telephoning. He tried hard to telephone, he tried hard to get the connection. The wires seemed to be cut, however, and he grew puzzled, and knit his brows and swore, and tried again and again, over and over."[154] His desperation to make the connection grows while the pointless surgery continues until the man triumphantly proclaims from the depths of delirium, "*Ça y est maintenant! Ça y est! C'est le bon Dieu à l'appareil!* (All right now! All right! It is the good God at the telephone!)."[155] This desperate and failed attempt to communicate by a dying man comes to naught, but the nurse can bring his final moments to the page where she and the reader stand as witnesses to his life and death.

This event made a significant impression on at least three people who witnessed it. In addition to La Motte writing about it, Warner recounted her version of the patient's story in a speech, describing "the boy field telephonist who thought his oxygen treatment was more telephoning, and said as he died that God was at the other end of the line."[156] Clapp returned to it as well in a chapter of *A Green Tent in Flanders*, "Ward I. The Telephone." In a deliberate rewriting of La Motte's text she provides a more human face to this patient; she too says he is a boy, "a beautiful boy," not the married man of La Motte's story, who, under the effects of the spinal, raves about his wife, but a young man of twenty with "a thick crop of black hair worn rather long, and dark, languid eyes."[157] He does not have a wound; rather, he is terribly ill with "typhoid fever and appendicitis."[158] Joined by his father and uncle, "for six lagging weeks the sympathy and science of the hospital clung to the chance of saving him, of saving those three lives," a more sympathetic and hopeful portrait than the one painted by La Motte.[159] His end, however, remains the same, with his fretting about making contact with his comrades to tell them urgently that "The Germans are coming! They come! They come! *Sauvez vous, camarades! Les boches sont là ... Allô.* No. 129?" before dying after commenting, "*Ah, ca y est, maintenant. Le bon Dieu est à l'appareil.*"[160] The addition of the "*ah*" and the use of periods instead of exclamations communicates a sense of calm sadness for the end of his confused final state. While he faces the same fate, death, as the man at the center of La Motte's story, he is surrounded by family and in the competent and caring embrace of the hospital.

La Motte would return to the necessity of acting as a "ghost writer" poignantly in "The Interval" when the nurse describes one dying patient: "He wants to write ... He has a block of paper and a pencil, and all day long he writes ... he gives the paper to every one who passes. He's got something on his mind that he wants to get across, before he dies. But no one can understand him. No one can read what he has written–it is just scrawls, scribbles, unintelligible."[161] On their own, the writings of this dying soldier are incomprehensible scratches: evidence of a desire to communicate, but also a sign of that impossibility. The pain that scribbling and scrawls mask remains unarticulated–conveying no comprehensible message any more successfully than the screams and moans of her patients filling the nurse's ears. Though the nurse can neither read the scribbled message, nor decipher her patients' cries, she can expand her role as intermediary by combining the functions of nurse and artist, thus ensuring that the reader hears the unintelligible sound of forgotten anonymous soldiers. She does not have the ability to render literally the meaning of those indecipherable signs, but she does have the power to attest to their existence.

The story also returns to another common thread in *The Backwash of War*: the concept of the "interval." The narrator comments, "death is dignified and life is dignified, but the intervals are awful. They are ludicrous, repulsive."[162] This observation comes after describing the slow and terrible deaths of several patients in the ward, those who are condemned to inhabit this "interval" where "they are gross, absurd, fantastic" before being liberated by the finality and cleanliness of death.[163] This space is similar in concept to the "backwash" described by La Motte in the introduction as "a stagnant place … [where] there is much ugliness."[164] The effects of working and living in this stifling liminality where patients hover between life and death and the ugliness of human suffering took their toll on La Motte and she left the hospital toward the end of February, suffering from a bad cold–although Mortimer was sure she was exaggerating her condition in order to leave the hospital.[165] By mid-March she was vacationing once again in Spain with Emily Chadbourne. She returned for a short stint at the hospital in May 1916 and then in early July she returned to New York City on *La Touraine*, landing at Ellis Island to spend some time in the United States visiting family in New York and Chicago and preparing for her next voyage. This time she would turn away deliberately from western Europe, the place that had served as her home and fostered her creative work for the past three years, to travel east.

Notes

1 Private Collection, Ellen N. La Motte, Unpublished Diary (hereafter Diary), "August 17, 1915."
2 Christine E. Hallett, "Portrayals of Suffering: Perceptions of Trauma in the Writings of First World War Nurses and Volunteers," *Canadian Bulletin of Medical History / Bulletin canadien d'histoire de la médicine* 27:1 (2010), p. 74.
3 In "Portrayals of Suffering," Hallett discusses how trained nurses and volunteers alike often provided "vivid descriptions of their patients' wounds," perhaps as a reaction to "the extraordinary nature of the wounds themselves," the heretofore unknown consequences of "industrial warfare," p. 72.
4 La Motte, Diary, "July 18, 1915."
5 For more information about the hospital and a broader perspective on its workings and medical staff, see Christine E. Hallett, *Nurses of Passchendaele: Caring for the Wounded of the Ypres Campaigns 1914–1918* (Barnsley, South Yorkshire: Pen & Sword, 2017).
6 La Motte, Diary, "July 18, 1915."
7 Margaret H. Darrow, *French Women and the First World War: War Stories of the Home Front: The Legacy of the Great War* (Oxford: Berg, 2000), p. 139.
8 La Motte, Diary, "July 19, 1915."
9 *Ibid.*

10 *Ibid.*, "July 20, 1915."
11 *Ibid.*, "July 23, 1915."
12 La Motte treated Esmeralda as a pet, letting her on her bed, taking photos of her, and showering her with affection. Her enthusiasm for her was not shared by many of the other hospital staff, who understandably resented her intrusion into the various *salles*. La Motte was forced to part with her when one of the night-duty nurses threatened to leave the hospital after being repeatedly woken by Esmeralda, explaining "night duty is sufficiently arduous without having it made worse by the selfish caprices of other nurses." La Motte "did not wish to make it hard for Mrs. T so gave poor little 'Esmy' to one of the laundry women." See La Motte, Diary, "September 25, 1915." While La Motte does not record "Esmy's" fate in her diary, in the 1934 edition of *The Backwash of War* she added one story in which after the narrator gives her "precious, beloved little goat" away, she discovers she has provided "a delicious meal" to the laundry woman who took her in. See E. La Motte, "Esmeralda," in *The Backwash of War* (New York: G. P. Putnam's Sons, 1934), p. 204.
13 La Motte, Diary, "July 23, 1915."
14 *Ibid.*, "July 24, 1915."
15 *Ibid.*
16 *Ibid.*, "July 25, 1915."
17 *Ibid.*, "July 26, 1915."
18 Christine E. Hallett, *Nurse Writers of the Great War*, Nursing History and Humanities (Manchester: Manchester University Press, 2016), p. 78.
19 Katrin Schultheiss, *Bodies and Souls: Politics and the Professionalization of Nursing in France, 1880–1922* (Cambridge, MA: Harvard University Press, 2001), p. 146.
20 *Ibid.*, p. 151.
21 *Ibid.*
22 La Motte, Diary, "August 20, 1915."
23 See C. E. Hallett, *Veiled Warriors: Allied Nurses of the First World War* (Oxford: Oxford University Press, 2014), p. 25.
24 La Motte, Diary, "August 7, 1915."
25 *Ibid.*
26 La Motte, Diary, "August 8, 1915."
27 Schultheiss explains that one of the conditions medical professionals put on the use of women as nurses in military hospitals was that nurses subordinate themselves absolutely to the authority of doctors. See *Bodies and Souls*, p. 151. Clearly, Borden Turner was not abiding by this expectation when she questioned the French doctor's choices and reported him to his superiors.
28 La Motte, Diary, "August 11, 1915."
29 *Ibid.*, "August 12, 1915."
30 *Ibid.*, "August 13, 1915."
31 *Ibid.*

32 *Ibid.*
33 *Ibid.*
34 *Ibid.*, "July 25, 1915."
35 *Ibid.*, "September 1, 1915."
36 Born Maude Ede, she published "Behind the Yser" and *A Green Tent in Flanders* under the name Maud Mortimer, though her married name was Maud Mortimer Clapp.
37 Ellen N. La Motte, "Heroes," *Atlantic Monthly* 118:2 (August 1916), p. 208.
38 *Ibid.*, p. 209.
39 FMCP "Ellen N. La Motte to Maud Mortimer Clapp," August 29, 1915.
40 La Motte, "Heroes," p. 208.
41 *Ibid.*, p. 209.
42 *Ibid.*, p. 210.
43 *Ibid.*
44 *Ibid.*
45 *Ibid.*
46 *Ibid.*
47 Hallett describes how many nurses' writings articulated their experiences within a heroic narrative mode to demonstrate the sacrifices they made doing important and potentially dangerous work during the war. See Hallett, *Veiled Warriors*, pp. 10–16. Undoubtedly, what made La Motte's story objectionable to many was its resistance to casting nursing in that mode in "Heroes."
48 " 'The Contributors' Column–September *Atlantic*,'" *Atlantic Monthly* 118:3 (September 1916).
49 " 'The Contributors' Column–November *Atlantic*,'" *Atlantic Monthly* 118:5 (November 1916).
50 *Ibid.*
51 See Chapter 3 for a more prolonged discussion of the article.
52 Frank H. Mason, "The American Ambulance," *Survey* 34:25 (September 1915), p. 563.
53 *Ibid.*
54 *Ibid.*
55 See Chapter 3 for discussion of her forays into fiction writing before the war.
56 Private Collection, "G. P. Putnam's Sons to Mary E. Lent," June 15, 1916.
57 Private Collection, "George H. Putnam to E. N. La Motte," July 19, 1916.
58 *Ibid.*
59 Launched in 1911, the *Masses* was a socialist journal founded by Piet Vlag that flourished under the editorial leadership of Max Eastman until it was forced to cease publication in 1917, when the United States government barred it from being circulated via mail. See the Modernist Journals Project (http://modjourn.org/render.php?view=mjp_object&id=MassesCollection) for a brief overview and PDFs of the journal. Undaunted, Eastman, with his sister, began publishing the *Liberator* in 1918. Like the *Masses*, it was socialist

in orientation. The Eastmans ceased to act as editors in 1922, and the journal ended its run in 1924. PDF copies are available at the Marxists Internet Archive (https://marxists.org/history/usa/culture/pubs/liberator/).

60 Max Eastman, *Love and Revolution: My Journey through an Epoch* (New York: Random House, 1964), p. 72.

61 W.G. Fuller, "The Lady with the Lamp," *Masses* 9:3 (January 1917), p. 30.

62 Floyd Dell, "The Book of the Month," *Masses* 9:3 (January 1917), p. 30.

63 For more about these women and Heterodoxy, see J. Schwarz, *Radical Feminists of Heterodoxy: Greenwich Village 1912–1940* (Norwich, VT: New Victoria Publishers, 1986). A scrapbook, "Heterodoxy to Marie," contains the photos and signatures of a number of members, including La Motte. See Inez Haynes Irwin Papers, 1872–1945 (hereafter IHIP), Schlesinger Library, Radcliffe Institute, Harvard University, Cambridge, MA. See Chapter 5 for more discussion of her connection to this group.

64 La Motte, Diary, "July 28, 1915."

65 Private Collection, "Edward Putnam to Ellen N. La Motte," July 19, 1916.

66 La Motte, Diary, "September 24, 1915."

67 FMCP, "Agnes Warner to Maud Mortimer Clapp," January 13, 1916. The letter is dated 1916 but undoubtedly should be 1917, after La Motte's book was published and Mortimer had finished working in the hospital.

68 Private Collection, "Edward Putnam to Ellen N. La Motte," July 31, 1917.

69 *Ibid.*

70 See Chapter 5 for a discussion of censorship of the book.

71 FMCP, "Maud Mortimer Clapp to Belle Clapp," November 17, 1913. The woman who "gave" La Motte to the Clapps is not clear; "Tim" is Frederick Mortimer Clapp, Maud Mortimer's husband.

72 FMCP, "Maud Mortimer Clapp to Frederick Mortimer Clapp," May 25–26, 1915.

73 *Ibid.*

74 *Ibid.*

75 FMCP, "Ellen N. La Motte to Maud Mortimer Clapp," July 15, 1915.

76 FMCP, "Ellen N. La Motte to Maud Mortimer Clapp," August 29, 1915.

77 *Ibid.*

78 See the entry in *Encyclopedia of American Biography*, vol. 32 (New York: American Historical Society, 1963), pp. 214–216, for more information about Clapp. The biography states she was born in Constantinople, whereas she says in *A Green Tent in Flanders* that she was born in Budapest; see Maud Mortimer, *A Green Tent in Flanders* (New York: Doubleday, 1917), p. 24.

79 The Frick Collection Records of the Organizing Director–Frederick Mortimer Clapp, 1920–1937, Frick Art Reference Library, New York, "Historical Note, Finding Aid."

80 FMCP, "Maud Mortimer Clapp to Mrs. W. F. Clapp," August 11, 1912.

81 FMCP, "Ellen N. La Motte to Maud Mortimer Clapp," November 11, 1915.

82 *Ibid.*
83 *Ibid.*
84 Mortimer, *A Green Tent*, p. 19.
85 La Motte, Diary, "June 19, 1915."
86 FMCP, "Maud Mortimer Clapp to Frederick Mortimer Clapp," December 11, 1915.
87 FMCP, "Maud Mortimer Clapp to Frederick Mortimer Clapp," November 16, 1915.
88 Diary, "October 3, 1915."
89 FMCP, "Maud Mortimer Clapp to Frederick Mortimer Clapp," January 4, 1916.
90 *Ibid.*
91 FMCP, "Maud Mortimer Clapp to Frederick Mortimer Clapp," January 17, 1916.
92 See Janet S.K. Watson, "Wars in the Wards: The Social Construction of Medical Work in First World War Britain," *Journal of British Studies* 41:4 (October 2002), pp. 484–510.
93 FMCP, "Maud Mortimer Clapp to Frederick Mortimer Clapp," January 19, 1916.
94 FMCP, "Maud Mortimer Clapp to Frederick Mortimer Clapp," January 28, 1916.
95 *Ibid.*
96 FMCP, "Maud Mortimer Clapp to Frederick Mortimer Clapp," February 1, 1916.
97 *Ibid.*
98 FMCP, "Maud Mortimer Clapp to Frederick Mortimer Clapp," January 28, 1916.
99 *Ibid.*
100 FMCP, "Maud Mortimer Clapp to Frederick Mortimer Clapp," February 9, 1916.
101 *Ibid.*
102 FMCP, "Maud Mortimer Clapp to Frederick Mortimer Clapp," February 12, 1916.
103 *Ibid.*
104 *Ibid.*
105 *Ibid.*
106 FMCP, "Maud Mortimer Clapp to Frederick Mortimer Clapp," February 16, 1916.
107 FMCP, "Maud Mortimer Clapp to Frederick Mortimer Clapp," February 20, 1916.
108 Watson, "Wars in the Wards," p. 503.
109 FMCP, "Maud Mortimer Clapp to Frederick Mortimer Clapp," February 23, 1916.

110 *Ibid.*
111 Mortimer, *A Green Tent*, p. 27.
112 *Ibid.*, pp. 27–28.
113 *Ibid.*, p. 156.
114 *Ibid.*, p. 157.
115 *Ibid.*
116 *Ibid.*, p. 183.
117 Ellen N. La Motte, "Pour la Patrie," in *The Backwash of War* (New York: G. P. Putnam's Sons, 1916), pp. 115–116. Subsequent quotations are from this edition unless otherwise noted.
118 La Motte, "Introduction," *The Backwash of War*, p.vi.
119 FMCP, Maud Mortimer Clapp, Unpublished Diary, "January 26, 1916."
120 La Motte, "Women and Wives," *The Backwash of War*, p. 105.
121 *Ibid.*, p. 98.
122 *Ibid.*, p. 99.
123 *Ibid.*, p. 100.
124 *Ibid.*, pp. 101–102.
125 *Ibid.*, p. 103.
126 *Ibid.*, p. 106.
127 *Ibid.*
128 See Chapter 2 for a discussion of La Motte's work in this capacity.
129 La Motte, "Women and Wives," *The Backwash of War*, p. 107.
130 *Ibid.*, pp. 107–108.
131 See Chapter 3 for discussion of the article.
132 La Motte, Diary, "July 26, 1915."
133 *Ibid.*, "July 27, 1915."
134 La Motte, "A Belgian Civilian," *The Backwash of War*, p. 63.
135 *Ibid.*, p. 64.
136 *Ibid.*, p. 66.
137 *Ibid.*, p. 67.
138 *Ibid.*, pp. 69–70.
139 *Ibid.*, p. 73.
140 La Motte, "A Citation," *The Backwash of War*, p. 168.
141 *Ibid.*
142 *Ibid.*, pp. 169–170.
143 *Ibid.*, p. 172.
144 *Ibid.*, pp. 174–175.
145 *Ibid.*, p. 176.
146 *Ibid.*, p. 178.
147 La Motte, "La Patrie Reconnaissante," *The Backwash of War*, p. 20.
148 *Ibid.*, p. 21.
149 La Motte, "Alone," *The Backwash of War*, p. 57.
150 *Ibid.*

151 *Ibid.*, p. 58.
152 *Ibid.*, p. 59.
153 La Motte, "At the Telephone," *The Backwash of War*, p. 159.
154 *Ibid.*, p. 162.
155 *Ibid.*, p. 163.
156 Shawna M. Quinn, *Agnes Warner and Nursing Sisters of the Great War* (Fredericton, New Brunswick: Goose Lane Editions, 2010), p. 146.
157 Mortimer, *A Green Tent*, p. 75.
158 *Ibid.*
159 *Ibid.*, p. 76.
160 *Ibid.*, pp. 76–77.
161 La Motte, "The Interval," *The Backwash of War*, pp. 89–90.
162 *Ibid.*, p. 91.
163 *Ibid.*, p. 87.
164 La Motte, "Introduction," *The Backwash of War*, p. v.
165 FMCP, Maud Mortimer Clapp, Unpublished Diary, "February 13, 1916."

5

The anti-opium crusade, 1916–1930s

La Motte's trek west from France to the United States, where she and Chadbourne visited friends and family before embarking for San Francisco,[1] the launching pad for their explorations of Asia, was noted in a dramatic short article, "Former Nurse is Seeking Respite from War's Roar," published in the *San Francisco Chronicle*. In it, the writer claimed that the two women were "on a tour of the world to recuperate from the nervous strain of long months of service in hospitals on the battlefields of France."[2] La Motte is cited as explaining that "As a result of the continuous rattle and roar of the artillery fire I became almost a nervous wreck," and La Motte and Chadbourne viewed travel as "good for [their] nerves,"[3] casting them as highly wrought, damaged by the war, and in need of healing through exploration.

However, as early as July 1915 Emily Chadbourne was thinking of going to China, commenting in a letter to Gertrude Stein that preferring "the Yellow Peril" to the war, she was going to invite La Motte to go to China with her when it was over.[4] She later placidly wrote to Stein that she spent her days doing "nothing" but they filled up all the same, representing her wartime experiences at that point as routine.[5] While critics have taken Stein's assessment of La Motte as "gun shy"[6] at face value,[7] La Motte's postcard to her mother from her third trip in May 1916 to Borden Turner's hospital remarks, "here I am back again, but this time the work is not hard, the weather is lovely, and I like it better!"[8] In the spring of 1916, the hospital had slowed down and the fighting shifted to the front on the Somme where Borden Turner established *L'Hôpital d'Evacuation* in the Sixth Army.[9] Although La Motte's final posting to the hospital, presumably a month-long stint similar to the one she served in January/February,[10] was, at least as represented to her mother, a calmer time than she had previously experienced, she had already begun to process her frontline nursing experiences in her fictionalized sketches. Whatever anger, frustration, and sadness she felt about what she did and observed in *L'Hôpital Chirurgical Mobile No. 1* was channeled into what would eventually constitute *The Backwash of War*, for which she signed the contract with G. P. Putnam's on July 28, 1916 in New York City, soon after her return from Europe, while she was visiting family and friends on the East Coast.[11] In the late summer and fall of 1916 more of her war writings were published: "Heroes" in August and "A Joy Ride: An Episode of Poperinghe" in October in the *Atlantic Monthly* and *The Backwash of War* by Putnam's, also in the fall. By the end of September, the Baltimore *Evening Sun*, whose readers would have been familiar with La Motte from her years of tuberculosis work and suffrage activity in the city, had reviewed the book, commenting that "those who volunteer, unasked, to minister to their [patients'] final sufferings [should] keep silence concerning the experiences … it is regrettable that these depths [of suffering] should be recorded other than in hospital records."[12]

After the entry of the United States into World War One in April 1917, the official view of La Motte's book would be that it was indeed "regrettable" that she had ever written it. In August 1917, the postmaster of Chehalis, WA, Elmer McBroom, undoubtedly encouraged by the Postmaster General's invitation in June 1917 to all local postmasters to keep a "close watch on unsealed matter, newspapers, etc., containing matter which is calculated to interfere with the success of any Federal loan … or to cause insubordination, disloyalty, mutiny, or refusal of duty in the military or naval service, or to obstruct the recruiting, draft, of enlistment services … or otherwise embarrass or hamper the Government in conducting the war,"[13] wrote to the solicitor of the United States Post Office in Washington, DC that he had seized books and pamphlets that a citizen had attempted to mail, one of which was La Motte's *Backwash of War*.[14] The acting solicitor, J. J. Southerland, responded a week later with a request that the items be held from the mail while an investigation was undertaken.[15]

The status of her book seems to have been left unresolved until a much more insistent writer, Robert Adger Bowen, with the Office of the Postmaster in New York City, contacted William H. Lamar, solicitor of the Post Office Department, in May of 1918. He excoriated La Motte's book, stating that "it would be difficult for either the author of this most depressing and repulsive book, or for the publishers, to give any valid reason for its appearance at this time."[16] Like many other critics, he took issue with its unrelentingly negative depiction of the hospital and its inhabitants and lambasts her for "rubbing in, the most loathsome physical manifestations of a hospital for the desperately wounded, and in that respect there are passages that are obscene in their realism–since this is not a medical treatise."[17] Further condemning the text, he levels harsh criticism at what he sees as "a cynical judgment of everything, including the hospital work even to its surgery and comprising the war itself, which cannot but reach [*sic*] unfavorably upon the average reader."[18] He concludes by "urgently advis[ing] its immediate suppression."[19]

Bowen's reading is surprisingly detailed given its bureaucratic origin. Bowen, however, studied at the College of Charleston and Washington and Lee University before completing some graduate work in English at Cornell University, which he left to begin working in publishing in New York City and to launch his own career as a writer.[20] After more than twenty years he joined the federal government at the beginning of World War One.[21] In his own telling, shared in the pages of the *Greenville News* during the 1930s, "there was established in the general postoffice [*sic*] in New York a federal bureau to function under the espionage and trading with the enery [*sic*] acts. Its duty was, through its staff of some 45 translators, many of them post office employees … to examine for seditious utterances every foreign language publication brought out in this country …. In addition, all English language printed material passing though the New York mail … was read and, if need be, was reported upon by that bureau to the solicitor of the Postoffice department in Washington."[22] Bowen reports that after the end of the war, "the bureau was taken over by the United States Department of Justice," he was appointed director, and he named the office the Bureau of Translations and Radical Publications, the primary goal of which after the war was to root out communist activity and suppress the political activity of African American writers.[23]

Bowen undoubtedly had to do little convincing of Lamar, who requested that a search be made to see if *The Backwash of War* had previously been labeled "unmailable."[24] When no evidence could be found that it had been suppressed, he immediately moved that it be made so in a brief missive to Bowen.[25] Lamar had been collaborating with the Chief of the Bureau of Investigation during the war years on monitoring and suppressing anything construed as violating the Espionage Act of June 15, 1917.[26] Lamar's work, along with that of Postmaster General Albert S. Burleson and bureau director A. Bruce Bielaski, "yielded the first domestic surveillance program in the United States,"[27] and Bowen was eager to play his part in this assessment of the dangers of radical influences in and through literary texts. Their joint efforts resulted in the book's being unmailable until La Motte wrote repeatedly to Burleson after the end of war, requesting that the book no longer be suppressed and explaining that the sketches were "rather gruesome, but I had served a year in a field hospital, and one could not help being affected by the tragedies of it all."[28] She received a reply several weeks later telling her that "the Postmaster at New York has been directed to accept copies of your book."[29] La Motte was fortunate that the ban was lifted as early as it was: the *Masses*, founded by Max Eastman, was labelled unmailable in the summer of 1917 and its mailing privileges would not be reinstated until August 1920, and then against Burleson's will–he had refused to lift the ban against the publications he had named as unmailable during the war years.[30] Given the praise heaped on *The Backwash of War* by the writers of the *Masses*,[31] it was fortuitous that Lamar relented and allowed the book to be recirculated as early as at the end of 1918.

This suppression and condemnation all lay in the future for La Motte. In the summer of 1916, she escaped the war, Europe, and the censure that her writing about the war brought her way by turning her attention to her travels.[32] She visited Colorado on her way to California, then Hawaii, before embarking for Japan.[33] She and Chadbourne landed in Japan by mid-September and spent six weeks traveling before going to Peking via Korea.[34] The women became enthralled by the intrigues and politics in the city and stayed until the end of November. With the onset of cold weather, they departed for Cambodia, the reason for which they had gone to Asia originally.[35] From there, they traveled to Thailand and Singapore, where La Motte applied for an extension to her passport. They returned to Peking in March of 1917 after a three-month absence and allowed themselves another month or so before they returned to Japan to see the cherry blossoms in April and stayed until June 1917. By summer, the two women were back in New York City, approximately a year after they had left.

During these months of travel, La Motte underwent an immersive education in the origins and consequences of the opium trade. On her way to Japan, she met Taraknath Das, an anti-British revolutionary from Bengal, India. When La Motte met him in 1916, he had been agitating on behalf of Indian independence at least since the highly controversial partitioning of Bengal in 1905. He spent time in the United States working for the cause, founding the *Free Hindusthan*, "an organ of freedom, and of political, social and religious reform,"[36] and enrolling in Norwich University, the oldest private military college in the United States, where he studied engineering and undoubtedly hoped "to obtain military training."[37] He was "honorably discharged"[38] from the university for continuing to agitate against Great Britain but eventually earned a B.A., M.A., and Ph.D. from American universities and became an American citizen.[39] In *The Opium Monopoly*, La Motte refers to meeting "a young Hindu"–though unnamed he must be Das–who roused them out of their ignorance regarding the deadly consequences of British opium policies by being "outspoken and indignant over the British policy of establishing the opium trade in India … Of all the phases of British rule in India, it was this policy which excited him the most" because "he greatly deplored the slow, but steady demoralization of the nation which was in consequence taking place."[40] La Motte and Chadbourne were incredulous as they learned "That such conditions existed," especially "in this age, with the consensus of public opinion sternly opposed to the sale and distribution of habit-forming drugs."[41] They were "So shocked … by what this young Hindu told us, that we flatly refused to believe him. We listened to what he had to say on the subject, but thinking … he must be mistaken … We decided not to take his word for it, but to look into the matter for ourselves."[42]

Das' biographer adds more details to the picture of the encounter: according to him, they met on the *Tenyo Maru* en route to Japan. Das facilitated discussions on the deck of the boat, and La Motte and Chadbourne "asked him 'a thousand questions, which he was pleased to answer.' "[43] Mukherjee also asserts that the three "met

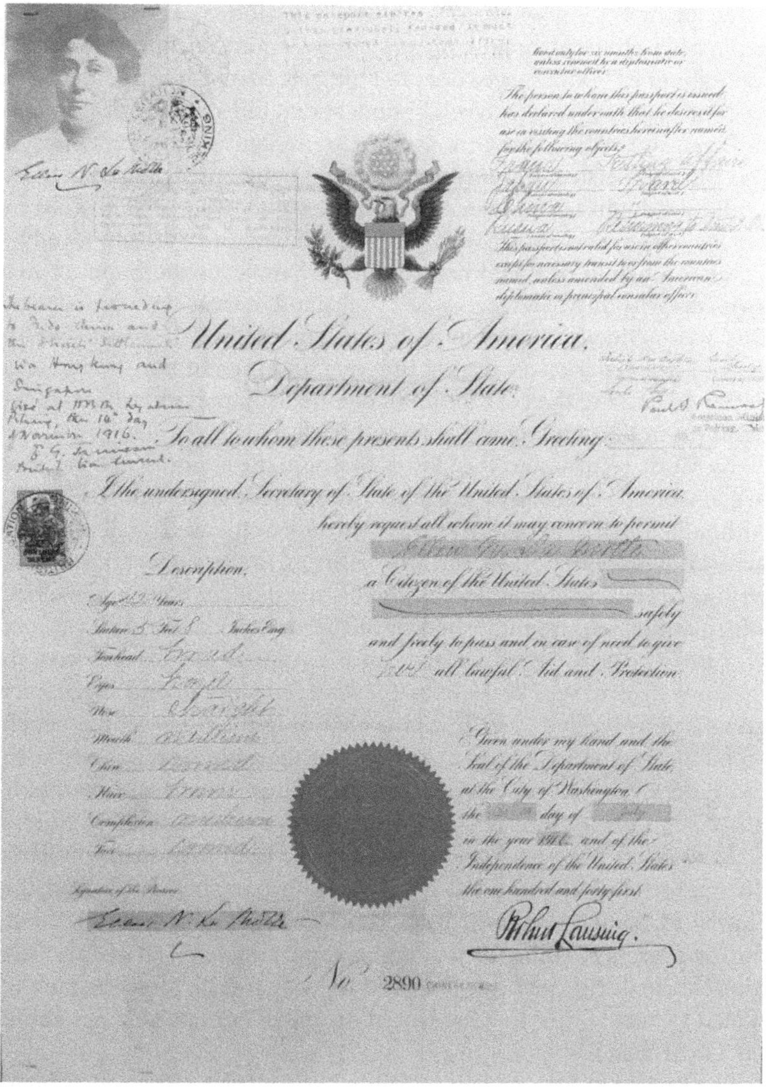
United States of America.
Department of State.
To all to whom these presents shall come, Greeting:
I the undersigned, Secretary of State of the United States of America,
hereby request all whom it may concern to permit
a Citizen of the United States
safely
and freely to pass and in case of need to give
all lawful Aid and Protection.
Description.
Given under my hand and the
Seal of the Department of State,
at the City of Washington
in the year
and of the
Independence of the United States
the one hundred and forty-first.
No. 2890

Figure 8 La Motte's passport, 1916–1917

… again in Peking where [Das] drew [La Motte's] attention to the deplorable effect of opium on the Chinese and encouraged her to write about it."[44] Mukherjee does not indicate that he was familiar with La Motte's previous substantial publications in the fields of nursing, suffrage, and World War One and may be assigning more influence to Das than is merited, but meeting a young, politically engaged activist would no doubt have resonated with La Motte, who, at this point in her life, was very familiar with actions, militant and not, employed to agitate on behalf of social justice causes. Whatever the impetus–her own curiosity and need to expose cruelty and injustice combined with Das' well-articulated critique of British colonialism–La Motte would harvest her experiences during this year and turn to non-fiction and fiction to explore the corruption of colonialism, particularly as it was manifest in the conduct of the opium trade.

La Motte returned to the United States in the summer of 1917 and began working on transforming her raw material into published texts. Although much of her creative energy would be focused on developing her writings about opium, she also returned to the subject of the war, writing several sketches, including "Esmeralda" in November 1917, which would not be published until the reissue of *The Backwash of War* in 1934, and "Without Jaws" and "Cripples," sketches written in the same cynical vein as those in *The Backwash of War* and that depict grievously wounded French soldiers sunning themselves on a bench on a busy boulevard where they contrast their physical injuries with those they call "moral cripples"–those who profited from or mindlessly supported the war.[45] She also wrote a draft sketch of Emma G. Mullen, an American who worked in the fashion industry in Paris during the war; she was killed when a German shell landed on the church of Saint-Gervais in Paris on Good Friday, March 29, 1918, during a service, killing or wounding approximately 150 people.[46] La Motte's friendship with her predated the war and La Motte began the sketch to "salute" her in what would be one of her last writings about the Great War.[47]

She turned to focusing on fulfilling her contract, which she signed on December 17, 1917, for *Peking Dust*, her first foray into writing about China in which she touches lightly on opium, and a conversational travel narrative in which she documented her experiences in Peking and reflected on the troubled relationship between the West and China. The book is addressed to an unnamed correspondent to whom she was prompted to write because she felt certain, after witnessing many injustices in China, that "some one else ought to know about it, too. Some one whose sense of justice had not become entirely warped."[48] She wrote letters she could never send because she "discovered all letters were opened" so she opted to collect them in a book along with articles from a variety of newspapers,[49] material that later became the substance of the book. The pretense in the book itself is that her correspondent, as she writes, "wanted me to tell you about our travels, particularly China,"[50] where she discovered "a surprising indifference to the results of the European war."[51] She explained this indifference as arising from the Chinese experience of "foreigners, saddening and enriching," which had resulted in the country being "a vassal state" and having "the curse of opium … forced upon her for commercial reasons."[52] This marks the first time La Motte wrote about the corruption of the opium trade, and in her usual blunt style she identified the problematic relationship between Europe and China, explaining:

> The structure of civilization that Europe has erected for itself is imposing and beautiful. We in America are confronted with the façade of this great building, and beheld from our side of the Atlantic it looks magnificent and superb. … But there is a back side to this structure of civilization; there are outbuildings, slums, and alleys not visible from the front. These back on the Orient, and the rear view of the structure of European civilization, seen from the Orient, is not imposing at all. The sweepings and refuse of Western Civilization and Western morality are dumped out upon the Orient, where they do not show.[53]

The language used in this passage echoes that of the introduction to *The Backwash of War*, in which La Motte describes the "many little lives foaming up in the backwash. They are loosened by the sweeping current, and float to the surface, detached from their environment …. By examining the things cast up in the backwash, we can gauge the progress of humanity."[54] La Motte delved into "the slime in the shallows" to reveal what she perceived as "weak, hideous, repellent" about human behavior during wartime.[55] In a similar move, she takes her correspondent and reader vicariously behind the "façade" of European civilization to investigate its "sweepings and refuse" to lay bare the hypocrisy of human behavior,[56] most pointedly the desire of "Western nations to keep this government in a state of weakness, of indecision, of susceptibility to bribes and threats; it makes China easier to control."[57] Her determination to probe beneath the surface to reveal the ugly and greedy side of human nature was renewed by her introduction to the realities of the long-term consequences of the opium trade in China and other nations under the control of Britain and a number of European countries.

The nature of the relationship between China and Westerners became more apparent to her as she traveled the country. She noted that "Americans, Europeans, foreigners of all sorts … always have the right of way, the privilege of walking over the Chinese, and to this privilege they must submit … due to a deep sense of fear of the consequences should they attempt to check or curb our activities or inclinations."[58] The result, she observes dryly, is "The relations between a subject people and their conquerors is fundamentally immoral and demoralizing to both."[59] This is particularly the case when the relationship is defined by the opium trade. La Motte describes how "Throughout China are the foreign concessions, small holdings of land which belong to the various European nations. … The Chinese have no authority or control over them, and are unable to regulate them in any way. … On Chinese soil the sale of opium is strictly prohibited; yet it is freely sold in foreign concessions, and the Chinese are powerless to prevent it."[60] For La Motte, this power imbalance was a revelation, one, after she had identified it, which would consume her for two decades as she learned about the origins of the opium trade, the immense profits earned by a number of colonial powers from it, and the devastating effects of the consequences of opium consumption and addiction.

Her education was furthered by being in Peking as the April 1, 1917 deadline, the date upon which China and Britain had agreed the opium trade would end, was quickly approaching. She read of attempts by the "Shanghai Opium Combine … to prolong the time limit for the sale of opium, to extend it for another nine months … because the combine has not sufficient time to sell off its remaining stocks of opium."[61] The solution to this excess of opium was for the Shanghai Opium Combine to induce "the Vice-President of China to purchase them in behalf of the Chinese government!"[62] La Motte condemns this deal as a "dastardly betrayal" and "a one-man deal" that the "Parliament and the country at large" responded to with "indignation."[63] The position of China was untenable: through the maneuverings of Feng Kuo Chang, the Vice President of China, the country was forced to pay $20 million for 3,000 chests of opium, becoming, just at the moment it was hoping to free itself from the trade, in effect a dealer of opium. Feng alleged that China could sell the opium for "medical purposes," but La Motte estimated it would take about "five hundred years" to unload such a quantity for legitimate reasons.[64] The result was the "humiliation" of China at the moment it should have been celebrating its release from the control of the British and the devastation of the opium traffic.[65]

La Motte witnessed additional gross attempts to manipulate China, this time by the Allies, in the same time period, trying to force it to break off diplomatic relations with Germany, which inevitably happened in August 1917, when China formally declared war. La Motte viewed this move as another example of China's manipulation at the hands of the West. In her interpretation, the origins of the war still raging in Europe emerged from "Supremacy in the Orient, control of the Far East–that is the underlying cause of the struggle which is rending Europe in twain."[66] China now was going to involve itself in a war, with all the sacrifice of people and resources that involved, waged in part to control it and its markets–a cruel twist to its long history of abuse and manipulation at the hands of European nations. As La Motte ruminates on the meaning of the war for China, she considers the discussion unfolding about memorializing the "five hundred Chinese soldiers" killed when the ship *Athos* was sunk in the Mediterranean by the Germans in February 1917.[67] One plan was to remove the inscription on the Ketteler Memorial in Peking, originally built to commemorate the death of Clemens von Ketteler, a German diplomat killed during the Boxer Uprising, and to rededicate it to the Chinese killed on the *Athos*. La Motte viewed this suggestion with cynicism, commenting that "It seems to me rather late in the day to begin inscribing pailows to Chinese killed by the conquering foreigner. … [it] leads one into sweeping vistas of all the pailows of China … all insufficient in their thousands to contain the names of the still greater thousands of Chinese slain by their European conquerors."[68]

Having had enough of the building tension and turmoil in Peking, she and Chadbourne decided to leave China on April 1, 1917 for

Japan. In some final thoughts, she mused that "We … are just about worn out with the strain on our sympathies. Opposition to a declaration of war is growing daily, and so are rumors of a revolution. … A revolution will offer the grand, final excuse for the 'protection' of China by Europe."[69] Anticipating that "European aggression or 'civilization' is the fate to which the Orient is predestined,"[70] they prepared to put some distance between themselves and potential violence. She asserted that "The World contains a double standard of international justice, for the East and the West" and that "With the attention of the world centered on Europe, things are taking place out here which could not possibly occur were the world free to know of them, and judge."[71] She returned to the imagery of the hidden ugliness lurking behind the European façade and asserted, "Back of the war, behind the war, ugly things are going on, which will be all finished and done with and safely accomplished by the time the war is over. The war for civilization is all that 'civilization' requires in the way of opportunity in the Orient."[72]

La Motte continued her meditation on the meaning of "civilization" in another book published in the same time period, spring 1919, as *Peking Dust*, this time a collection of short fiction, *Civilization: Tales of the Orient*, published with the George H. Doran Company. She returned to the form that had won her recognition with *The Backwash of War* and had success getting three stories published in advance in the *Century Magazine*, although her initial efforts to publish the stories as a collection were thwarted, she speculated in a letter to H. L. Mencken, because they "are awfully modern–too much so … for the modern reader."[73] Certainly, they take on a number of topics that would have been seen as controversial: the struggle of multiracial characters trying to find a sense of belonging, the abuse of Asians by their white "superiors," including economic exploitation and physical violence, and the loss of "civilized" values in Europeans living in Asia. Some reviewers saw these topics as too unrelentingly grim, echoing a similar criticism made about *The Backwash of War*, with one reviewer asserting that "she has allowed the land and its many tragedies to cloud her vision. And though her stories are well and brutally told, her desired effect is blunted by too much baseness. Unlike Burke, she can see no spark of goodness against which to draw her poignant contrasts."[74] Other reviewers had reservations but were more positive: the *Evening Sun* reviewer critiqued the collection because "In the way that Socialist literature often does, the case is made out too one-sided–most of us are pretty grey in character" but noted that the stories were "extremely well done–written with a particular kind of vigor which, a few years ago, would only have been described as masculine!"[75]

This ambiguous compliment may have been produced with stories like "The Yellow Streak," previously published in the *Century Magazine* in March 1919, in mind. It tackles the topic of sexuality and interracial identity through the character of Rogers, "a minor clerk in a big corporation" in Shanghai, at a time, "a generation ago … when [it] was not as respectable as it is now."[76] Rogers arrives at his post, "delicate and abstemious, and the East being new to him, shocked him."[77] He maintains his quiet ways, in contrast to most young men who arrive in the East, as the narrator tells us, explaining that life in the Far East "is generally stimulating and exciting, even to the most unimaginative, while the novelty of it, the utter freedom and lack of restraint and absence of conventional public opinion is that usually, within a very short time, one becomes unfitted to return to a more formal society."[78] Rogers surprises his compatriots when he too compromises his moral standards out of a strong desire for "a home of his own, a refuge to turn to at the end of each long monotonous day,"[79] and he begins "a partnership with a little Chinese girl who answered every purpose," including, unexpectedly, giving him a son.[80] Not having married, and not intending to stay in the East forever, Rogers is initially upset by this predictable development but comes to feel "in a vague way, fond of him" despite hating "half-breeds," who "are worse than the natives, having inherited the weakness of both ancestries."[81]

Rogers is able to escape the consequences of his decisions and actions when he is sent back to England after fifteen years, free to "find himself a home upon orthodox lines and live happily ever after afterwards."[82] Being "thoughtful and decent, far-sighted and provident," Rogers sends his wife back to her family and sets up financial support for her and his son, an act that enables him to feel smug and righteous as he leaves China, reflecting as he goes that "many men go to pieces out in the East, but he, somehow, had managed to keep himself clear and clean."[83] The ironic tone dominates this and most of the other stories in the collection; the narrator's barely concealed sarcasm disrupts the smug satisfaction of Rogers, who has been the main character up until this point. To underscore the self-deception of Rogers' interpretation of his actions, the narrator shifts the focus to the fallout of his actions: the fates of his Chinese partner and their son. She went "obediently back to the provinces, as had been arranged" and the "half-caste boy" was sent to school.[84] However, his memories of home and this pride in "his white blood" make him an outsider unable to find a sense of belonging with the Chinese or the Europeans.[85] As the narrator comments, "every one … knows the contempt that is shown a half-breed, a Eurasian. Neither fish nor fowl–an object of general distrust and disgust."[86]

The son cannot come to terms with his rejection from white society and wonders, "If his mother, pure Chinese, was good enough for his father, why was not he, only half-Chinese, good enough for his father's people?"[87] Striving to prove his worth, he is "exalted" when the war breaks out and he has the opportunity "to answer the call of the blood!"[88] Predictably, he never garners the respect and acceptance for which he searches through war service. Rather, returning an amputee on crutches with no one to greet him at the dock, he feels a new connection to "The great, brown, muddy Yangtzse,"[89] a connection he will need because nothing has changed in his absence: he sees "two young men … sleek, well-fed, laughing … old colleagues in the office" who "glanced in his direction, looked down on his pinned-up trouser leg, caught his eye, and then, without sign of recognition, passed on."[90] Ignored before the war, he remains ignored after the war–his absent leg neither a source of respect nor of compassion. The young white Englishmen who have harbored safely in China during the war feel no sense of obligation to him; "he was still a half-breed."[91]

Other stories in the collection explore additional corrupt power dynamics between Europeans and the Chinese. In "On the Heights," Rivers, an English "adventurer … and ne'er-do-weel …,"[92] sets up a hotel for Europeans in a Buddhist temple in an up-and-coming trade center in the interior. Like most of the European characters in La Motte's fiction, "Rivers had a profound contempt for the Chinese," which he demonstrated through "blows and curses as occasion required."[93] He takes particular pleasure in expressing his "contempt … for all those who had not his advantages–the great, God-given advantage of a white skin."[94] The hotel is eventually burned down in a revolution whose origins he does not understand, and Rivers counts on receiving compensation from the Chinese government for his losses. Despite receiving the money to rebuild his hotel, he seethes with bitterness and anger at the Chinese and takes great pleasure in cheating rickshaw drivers and beating workers, safe in the knowledge that "No coolie could successfully contradict the word of a foreigner … He was quite secure in his bullying, in his dishonesty, in his brutality, and there is no place on earth where the white man is more secure in his whitemanishness than in this Settlement, administered by the ruling races of the world."[95]

Even Rivers, however, is held to some small kind of accountability when he beats his former hotel worker, Kwong, who became an impoverished and ailing rickshaw driver in Shanghai, to death and has to stand trial. European "justice" is meted out and Rivers is "acquitted" and the cause of Kwong's death found to be "Accidental death due to rupture of the spleen, caused by over exertion."[96] Although Rivers is able to evade punishment, Kwong's son, "filled with an overmastering and bitter hatred of Rivers," takes justice into his own hands and obtains a job as a cook in Rivers' newly built hotel.[97] He waits until Rivers has successfully re-established himself then sneaks into his room, where he wakes Rivers up to enjoy the satisfaction of killing him, knowing Rivers was fully aware of his impending death and of being murdered at the hands of those he had abused and vilified. As Liu holds the knife at Rivers' throat, he "mounted to the heights" and "felt, for prolonged and glorious moments, the feelings of the superior race" before plunging the knife into him, thereby silencing permanently a cruel and despised man who had enjoyed wielding the power lent him by corrupt colonial power dynamics.[98]

Other stories in the collection are similarly concerned with exploring imperfect conceptions of justice. In "Homesick," Lawson, whose job it is to stop gambling in the Foreign Concession, stands with one foot on Chinese territory and one on land in the Concession, unable to pursue the owner of a gambling den because he has disappeared into Chinese territory. He muses, "Morality appeared arbitrary, determined by geographical lines …. What was right and wrong, anyway? What was moral or immoral, anyway?"[99] The narrator takes great pains to ensure the reader knows that Lawson is "of very limited intelligence," thus undercutting the import of his questions, which remain without answers and which Lawson abandons when given the opportunity to accept bribes to turn a blind eye to the gambling houses.[100] The money he accumulates will allow him to return home, though he has won that money at the cost of his ethics and of his interest in the injustice embedded in the ways laws are constructed and enacted. He can no longer question the meaning of the "arbitrary" nature of "morality" now that he has determined to use his position as an enforcer of laws to line his own pockets.

Like Lawson, other characters are able to escape punishment or the consequences of their immoral actions. In an egregious case, a "minor official in one of the colonies of his country," Mercier, fulfills one of his "romantic dreams" and moves to the "Tropics," a place he has imagined as "islands in southern seas, of unknown, mysterious life."[101] He is amazed by the beauty of the island, his new home and the location of the penal colony he is to oversee. It is "two days' sail from the nearest port on the mainland, the port itself ten thousand miles from home."[102] Inevitably, Mercier's enthusiasm dims when he meets the island's white inhabitants, who share their anxieties about escaping their posts to return home and their fatigue with the isolation of the island and their fear of poisonous insects. He quickly grows to despise one of the island's white inhabitants, a woman "aged, fat, and stupid,"[103] whose only positive quality is her daughter, "a child of perhaps fourteen"[104] to whom he is attracted for her imminent "blooming into womanhood."[105] The young girl, who suffers from an unnamed intellectual disability, has no hopes of marrying or being educated. She is a perfect, vulnerable target for his boredom and lust, and Mercier is certain that when their eyes met, the girl blushed as a result of feeling a "sensation, vague" and "shared."[106] Later, he sees the girl accompanied by "her body servant," a "Kling," a South Indian Muslim, and looking at her stretched out on the ground, he realizes she possesses a physically "mature" body and "A thought suddenly rose to his mind, submerging everything else."[107] He becomes obsessed by her body and goes so far as arguing with her mother to forbid her to roam the island with her servant because of the threat posed by the many convicts on the island, but of course, in reality "He had been pleading for protection against himself."[108] Unable to resist, and rationalizing that she felt "a note of passion–such as he felt for her," he rapes her on numerous occasions while the servant turns his back on the scene.[109] Eager to shift potential blame away from himself, he denounces the servant as a rapist, resigns his position, and leaves the island right after the servant is hanged. Like Rivers in "The Yellow Streak," he is able to exploit and abuse without consequences, while the vulnerable servant, who is implicated in the violence against the young girl by his silence, has to pay with his life.

In addition to placing European characters in Eastern settings, La Motte takes characters from the Far East and examines their fates when displaced to European countries. In "Civilization," she returns to World War One, only this time in her fiction, she focuses not on the world of the frontlines and hospitals, but on life in the civilian areas through the character of Maubert, the owner of a small wine shop and father of four children. Mobilized, despite being older and somewhat unfit, he has to leave his wife in charge of their business and family. He is abusive and angry that she refused to give him a fifth child, which would have shielded him from having to be called up for war service. Having no choice, he is sent to the front to serve as a sentry, a poor assignment for him since he is barely able to read the papers shown to him. He is eventually granted five days' leave, four of which will be taken up with traveling to and from his home in the provinces, but he only makes it as far as Paris, where, drunk, he fails to make his connection. He spends the rest of his leave satisfying himself with the prostitutes available in the Paris streets and never sees his wife and children.

Meanwhile, his wife, who has no reason to miss her violent and dull husband, is experiencing the other side of mobilization. As the narrator explains, "a further mobilisation of subjects of the French Empire was taking place" but "the forces were not mobilised but volunteered."[110] Repeating the words "volunteered," "volunteers," and "voluntarily," La Motte emphasizes the lack of choice Ouk, a citizen of the French Empire, has when he is forced to choose between serving as a volunteer to be sent to "civilization" or being punished for refusing to go by being sent to the jungle. He decides, "Of the two alternatives, the risks of civilization seemed preferable."[111] Thus, Ouk, along with hundreds of other men from the area, becomes familiar with "the ways of Europe … with difficulty and pain."[112] He is assigned to a munitions factory in Maubert's town where he eventually encounters Madame Maubert, whose bar he frequents, and "they realised, gazing at each other from opposite sides of the zinc covered bar, that Civilization claimed them. Each had a duty to perform towards its furtherance and enhancement."[113] At the very least, they further the species when she ends up bearing a fifth child after all, the very thing that will release Maubert from military service. He rages at her duplicity, seeing no contradiction in having spent his leave with prostitutes–the very period during which his wife was sleeping with Ouk. He cannot even avenge himself on Ouk, who, by this time, has died, as Madame Maubert explains, due to the damp and cold. Nevertheless, the fortuitous timing allows Maubert to lay claim to the child after accepting as a concession a baby that "looks like a Chinese" in order to guarantee his permanent release from wartime service.[114]

It is an interesting story that brings in discussions of nationalism, colonialism, and the value of wartime service only to dismantle them by showing how personal motivations and the promise of gain outweigh lofty external ideals. In this way, *Tales of the Orient* is similar to *The Backwash of War* and marks a thematic and stylistic continuity in her work. There is evidence too of her first professional preoccupations, public health concerns, in the collection. In the story "Cholera," she explores a cholera outbreak in Japan through the lens of class and contrasts the experience of foreigners and the Emperor with that of the working classes: the former group is fearful because they understand the deadly threat posed by the disease but the latter group is not because they "are ignorant" of its potential.[115] Meanwhile, on her travels in Asia, La Motte describes in *Peking Dust* how she was trying to throw off her own shackles and concerns about hygiene. Exploring the different sweets on offer at a bazaar she frequented in Peking, she describes the allure of the "sweet-stalls ... where wonderful Chinese candies and sugared fruits are for sale" and where she and Chadbourne "eat [their] way from stall to stall."[116] Stopping to consider the question of sanitation, she says:

> Germs? Maybe, but we don't care. I am sick of germs, of the emphasis that every one at home places on them. It's restful to get into a country where there aren't any, or at least people don't know about them. The trouble with America is that everyone is so busy thinking of clean streets, clean garbage-cans, the possibilities of impure food, that much of the beauty and comfort of life is lost. Life is not all in length.[117]

Although the comment is meant to be taken lightheartedly, it is telling that La Motte wanted to remove herself from the influence of the topic that had ruled her life both in Baltimore in the fight against tuberculosis and during the war in the hospital–the menace posed by germs and bacteria–in favor of a more carefree existence that threw caution to the wind.

If La Motte was trying to change her mindset deliberately, there is no doubt that her year of travels in Asia propelled her forward personally and professionally in significant ways. The story "Under a Wineglass" was first published in the *Century Magazine*, then in *Tales of the Orient*, and later selected for inclusion in *The Best Short Stories of 1919*, alongside works by Sherwood Anderson, Djuna Barnes, Susan Glaspell, and Anzia Yezierska, powerhouses of twentieth-century American writing. The story explores the significance of thwarted artistic ambition against the backdrop of the Gulf of Thailand. The story has Conradian elements, including the isolated setting, a steamer, and the suspension of activity that allows for the captain of the steamer to recount a story to a passenger about a man living in isolation on one of the islands in the gulf. The man, proclaimed a great artist after his first book is published, loses his artistic inspiration and capacity once he enters into a relationship with a rich woman he loves. It has the unintended consequence of "sapp[ing]" him of his "genius."[118] He initially does not mind the loss of inspiration, but he eventually feels as though there is an "intangible, transparent, strong wall, hemming him in, shutting in the gold."[119] The captain compares him to a statue of the Buddha over which "some one turned a wineglass" and who now "sits, still and immovable."[120] To break out and reclaim his voice, the man plots to leave his love despite being torn between "His life of happiness with her–[and] his work."[121] He eventually regrets his decision and desires to return to her, "Only now he was no longer gilded. He must gild himself anew, bright, just as she had found him."[122] His journey to find that "gilding" and a way to reclaim his art leads him to the isolation of an uninhabited island in the Gulf of Thailand where he lives in a hut and tries to produce his next great work; however, all comes to naught when he eventually dies alone, and the only text he has produced bears the word "Beloved."[123]

It is difficult not to draw parallels between the struggle of the main character and La Motte. She used her life experiences as the basis of her fiction and threaded autobiographical elements throughout her work, and like the man on the island, she had lived in the equivalent of a "garret in London, a studio off Montparnasse, shabby, hungry" before becoming involved with Chadbourne, a woman with financial resources that far exceeded her own.[124] Unlike the man in the story, she never left her partner to find artistic freedom but continued to write as she lived separately–maintaining her own more modest apartments over the years and frequently traveling without Chadbourne for long periods of time–but connected with her until their deaths in the 1960s. Perhaps for La Motte, preserving her independence financially and physically was enough to grant her the autonomy the man in the story feels has been taken from him despite he and his beloved genuinely loving each other. La Motte found a balance and maintained her personal freedom while building a relationship with a woman with whom she shared many interests, including art collecting, travel, and, to a degree, combating the opium trade.[125]

La Motte, the writer and experienced activist, took the public lead in becoming a vocal critique of the opium trade, but there are signs Chadbourne actively supported the cause and La Motte's activities on behalf of it. Certainly, La Motte used *Peking Dust* to explore her early understanding of the problem of opium in the relationship between the West and China and her fiction served as a vehicle for thinking through the devastation wrought by the drug. In "Canterbury Chimes" she depicts Bishop Herbert, a man of forty-five, stretched out enjoying the "climate of the Far Eastern Tropics" on his veranda when his reverie is disturbed by a poor native man who approaches him to appeal to him to take action against the opium trade.[126] The Bishop is insulted that the man would dare to challenge him by providing statistics regarding the buying and selling of opium and the enormous profits the colonizers make from ensuring natives are addicted to the drug. The man's education and clarity of speech are an affront to the Bishop, and he eventually attempts to strike him before he flees. The Bishop is rattled as a result and engages in a process of reflection and rationalization before deciding that it was "a matter for him to let alone."[127] Although he is a decent man, he cannot be bothered to cause disruption to his own peaceful and prosperous existence by taking up such a controversial cause. The next day his restored sense of tranquility is once again upset, this time by a letter from his brother communicating that his son is being sent out to stay with the Bishop to escape after committing a significant "dishonor."[128] The Bishop is as aghast at the prospect of this intrusion into his comfortable life as he was by the appearance of the young man who visited him the evening before. The Bishop anxiously awaits the steamer that will set his nephew loose on the island, where indulgences, such as easily available opium, will be difficult to resist. The nephew never appears, but eventually the Bishop is called to an opium den where a young man is dead after spending a week smoking. He fears the worst and is full of relief after determining that the young man is not his nephew.

The story investigates questions concerning exploitation and responsibility. The Bishop's life, which is mostly devoted to sensual pleasures such as eating, exercising, and relishing the weather, is supported by a salary, as the young man points out, that "comes from the established opium trade."[129] Yet, he never interrogates the cost of being able to enjoy his surroundings and privileges until he is unexpectedly challenged by the young man's facts and figures and the rightness, especially morally speaking, of his arguments. Motivated by a selfish desire to preserve his comfort, he sets aside these ugly realities and allows his racist perception of the man to guide his decision to disregard the encounter. The second interruption to his life, this time the threat that his nephew may be vulnerable to the corruption of the island, seems to shake his complacency, but it is unclear if the sight of the dead European man in the opium den is enough to provoke him to action. The bounty, for Europeans anyway, produced by opium profits is just too great for most to sacrifice it, no matter how morally bankrupt it is to live by such a problematic source of revenue.

It is on this point that La Motte would focus much of her energy in her writing devoted to the opium problem. She mustered all of her persuasive powers to try to communicate the threat posed by opium to public health and the absolute corruption of thriving financially when the very source of profits was a menace to so many millions of native people in colonized lands. This period, during which La Motte was honing her critiques of opium policy and writing *Peking Dust* and *Civilization: Tales of the Orient*, was one of adjustment and recalibration personally. At this point, she had lived abroad for the most part since June 1913, and her return to the United States marked the first time she was living there, since she first attended Johns Hopkins in 1898, as a writer and not a nurse.[130] She registered to vote in New York State "under the Republican Eagle,"[131] took up residence in the Buckingham Hotel on 5th Avenue and 50th Street, and used it as a base from which to work and promote her writings.

She and Chadbourne began making plans to return to Asia in the winter of 1917/1918, but they ran into difficulty obtaining passports. La Motte reached out to her cousin, Alfred I. du Pont, and asked him to use his influence with Senator Willard Saulsbury, Jr. of Delaware to help her and Chadbourne in securing them. Du Pont's response was a careful one: he explained that although he could use his connections to reach out on her behalf "as a personal favor … I would have to take upon myself the endorsement of everything that might result in consequence. While I am perfectly willing to take the responsibility as far as you are concerned, I could not do so with Mrs. Chadbourne, for I do not know her."[132] He cautiously added that "before such passports could be issued a very careful investigation would be made by the Secret Service Department, with a view to establishing so far as possible the unquestioned loyalty of both you and Mrs. Chadbourne to the United States, and if peradventure it should come to the ears of the State Department that either Mrs. Chadbourne or yourself had voiced a position of absolute neutrality, you may be sure that no passports would be issued, but on the contrary you would immediately be placed under surveillance, if nothing worse."[133]

She also asked her cousin, Thomas Coleman du Pont, to help in her quest, and the ensuing conversation preserved in records shows that in fact she and Chadbourne had been under some kind of surveillance. Du Pont made inquiries with the Attorney General, which led to a request by the "Chief," Bielaski, to Charles DeWoody, Division Superintendent of the New York Bureau of Investigation, to communicate with La Motte about her inquiry. According to his letter, La Motte had provided "information … to one of the men of your office … related to the Hindu case. General DuPont states that Miss LaMotte would like to know about the investigation but I believe she was interested in knowing whether or not the party she reported was all right."[134] It is unclear whom she reported and for what and whether or not Bielaski's suspicions were correct. In a follow-up, DeWoody informed Bielaski that an Agent Vander Poel had submitted a memo in April 1918 regarding the status of La Motte's passport and he met with her on May 8 about the same topic. DeWoody wrote that "She is laboring under the impression that the fact that she assisted a certain Hindu by the name of Taraknath Das ... prejudiced the State Department against her as a possible disloyal character."[135] The crux of the concern was that Chadbourne gave Das $10,000 toward bail and paid his attorney's fees when he was arrested in San Francisco for allegedly being involved in a plan to incite a rebellion against the British. DeWoody communicated that Vander Poel was "satisfied the women were perfectly innocent in the matter and that they are good loyal citizens of this country."[136] The Chief subsequently sent the head of the Bureau of Citizenship, R. W. Flouncy, a copy of DeWoody's letter, but if it was intended to clear the way for the issuance of passports, it did not have that result.

Other records show that the two women were being investigated as early as December 5, 1917, when letters from Chadbourne, La Motte, and Das were sent to John Lord O'Brian's assistant at the Department of Justice.[137] O'Brian oversaw the new War Emergency Division, which was responsible for enforcing the Espionage and Sedition Acts. Because of their correspondence, Winslow wrote, La Motte and Chadbourne were "put on the suspect list and interviewed by one of your agents."[138] It would take a request by Chadbourne's brother, Charles Crane, a businessman and politician, to L. Lanier Winslow of the Department of State to interview the two women to prompt further action. Winslow complied, meeting with them on May 14, 1919, and describing La Motte as "extremely clever and most interesting" and Chadbourne as "very rich."[139] He added, "I think it is a question of two lone women looking for a little excitement and adventure, with perhaps the romantic side of their natures a bit too far developed, coupled with an overabundance of money."[140] He remained noncommittal about whether or not they would be granted passports but assured O'Brian that "I feel they will be a little more careful in the near future. I gave them a long heart to heart talk and pointed out the error of their ways and how careful they should be and why they had gotten into all this trouble, and I think the next Indian or Hindu that approaches them will have a cold reception."[141]

The language of both DeWoody and Winslow is condescending toward La Motte and Chadbourne, middle-aged women in their forties that the men probably could not see as serious threats because of their age, gender, and class. Of course, they did not pose any threat to the safety of the United States, but DeWoody's statement that La Motte was "laboring under the impression that the fact that she assisted a certain Hindu by the name of Taraknath Das ... prejudiced the State Department against her as a possible disloyal character"[142] hints that she is delusional for believing such a charge could be brought against her. In fact, in September 1917, a lawyer with the British embassy in Washington, DC, Thomas Hohler, wrote to Leland Harrison at the Department of State to inquire if it "would ... be possible to decline to give them passports?" because of their "sympathy with certain Hindu propagandists, especially with an Taraknath Das."[143] Months earlier in May 1917, when La Motte and Chadbourne were still in Japan, C. J. Davidson, Vice-Consul in Yokohama, wrote to Conyngham Greene, the British ambassador to Japan, referring to earlier comments he had passed on about the women and underlining that he had "from the beginning suspected the relations of this woman [Emily Chadbourne] and her friend Miss La Matte [*sic*] with Tarak Nath [*sic*]."[144] Greene, in a letter to the Foreign Secretary, Arthur Balfour, seemed less inclined to agree with Davidson's concerns and conveyed that the American chargé d'affaires, Post Wheeler, attested that the women could not have had any knowledge of Das' revolutionary activities or of the warrant issued for his arrest in the United States.[145]

Greene's next dispatch to Balfour, however, sent only five days later, reversed course and claimed that the women were "reported to have given utterance to violently anti-British sentiments during their stay at Tokyo, and to have deplored the entry of their country into the war on the side of the Allies."[146] He emphasized that Davidson was "firmly persuaded that these ladies are fully aware of Tarak Nath's true character ... and that they have not subscribed to the funds of the Hindustan Association of America under a mistaken conception of its aims."[147] Reports submitted by two agents were used to confirm the purportedly nefarious relationship between them: Agent S. verified that La Motte and Chadbourne left Japan for San Francisco on June 5 and, in an attempt to belittle Das, claimed that he "went to see them off from Yokohama. He busied himself looking after their baggage, etc, behaving as if he were their servant."[148] He further elaborated that one of the women gave Das "about 300 Yen, and as the ship left the wharf the two ladies and Dass [*sic*] continued to wave their handkerchiefs to one another."[149]

Several days later, Agent P. filed a longer report on La Motte, Chadbourne, and Das, asserting that "They [the women] are going to do something in the way of helping the Indians under trial in America. It is also likely that they may give financial help to the revolutionary movement in America."[150] These speculative official reports were followed up by some gossip: Greene shared with Balfour that "a United States citizen, who made the journey from Bordeaux with these two ladies states that the latter is the author of a work entitled 'Backwash of War' in which she severely criticizes French military hospitals and that this has aroused great indignation in France."[151] In this case, the gossip was quite accurate given the reaction to the book of those who worked in the hospital with her.[152] The next statement, however, undercuts his informant's reliability. In one simple sentence, Greene says, "He regards Mrs. Chadbourne as slightly deranged."[153] Others also were concerned about Chadbourne's state of mind. Richard Gottheil, a scholar in Woods Hole, MA, who knew Chadbourne's brother, Charles Crane, wrote after seeing Chadbourne not long after her return to the United States that Chadbourne was "pro-German" and "anti-English" because of the "anti-opium matter."[154]

The fact that La Motte, Chadbourne, and Das continued to correspond after the women left Japan led to their mail being intercepted, examined, and interpreted to decipher any malevolent intent, which the British certainly located in their correspondence. One writer from the British embassy claimed that they had "considerable power for evil" because they were suspected of "arranging for the publication of anglophobe literature in the United States."[155] In one such intercepted letter, Das wrote to Chadbourne about manuscripts that "must be published, if it is at all practicable."[156] He also explained that "As the Japanese translation of my small book has been suppressed by the authorities for reasons best known to them … it will depend upon you and Miss L. to get a publisher for the work."[157] A month later, La Motte confirmed to Das that she had "all the mss. now–it came safely, but the last parts I did not use, I thought it was superfluous, and the book as I have written it, does not seem to need anything more. All is said, anyway, and excellently said too, if do [*sic*] have to say so myself. At present it is in the hands of a first class publisher here."[158] It is not clear which manuscripts Das had sent them and how La Motte was supposed to integrate them into *Peking Dust*,[159] but some kind of potential collaboration between them had been arranged. The potential ramifications of such collusion could have been very serious for La Motte. In a letter to Major Thwaites with the British Military Mission in New York, "N." made the serious claim that:

> Miss La Motte brought into the United States the English manuscript of Taraknath Das' violent anti-American and anti-English pamphlet, "The Isolation of Japan in World Politics." Taraknath Das and Agnes Brundin of New York have been indicted under the sedition act for attempting to publish this noxious work in the United States. It seems to me very likely that Miss La Motte also made herself criminally liable for her participation in this affair.[160]

La Motte was either protected by the influence of the du Pont family, or further evidence materialized that she had not transported the text to the United States. Das was arrested, as was Agnes Smedley, the real name of Agnes Brundin, "for attempting to stir up rebellion against British rule in India."[161] Smedley was caught with copies of "The Isolation of Japan in World Politics" that she was disseminating, damning evidence of her belief in and support for Indian independence. Whether she somehow received copies of that text because La Motte brought it into the United States is uncertain but unlikely, given that La Motte would have faced much closer scrutiny and charges had she done so.

La Motte seems to have had faith in Das' innocence: she wrote to him in August 1917, in another letter intercepted by the British authorities, that he should "come to America if necessary, and have the chance to clear yourself, and let us know the minute you get here. Remember that you have two good friends who have great faith in you, and who will do everything to help you out of the difficulty."[162] La Motte did not know that Das had, according to the American embassy in Tokyo, already left Japan for the United States earlier in the month.[163] Wheeler's letter explains that Das asserted his innocence and requested reimbursement for his travel costs since he was compelled to go to the United States to clear his name. He ended up being arrested upon arrival in San Francisco, tried with a large group of other men, and sentenced to twenty months in prison. Although he might have blamed La Motte for encouraging him to return to face certain arrest, he apparently did not. Imprisoned in Leavenworth in Kansas, Das continued his writing and "study of politics, philosophy and religion, arts, and literature."[164] He asked a lawyer, Charles Recht, for help publishing a manuscript in pamphlet form and wanted it to be dedicated "to E & E."[165]

One can only imagine that the two women would have been loath to attract attention in 1918, when they were still having difficulty obtaining passports, by being associated with a convicted revolutionary, and no evidence has surfaced that the dedication made it into print. Das also acknowledged La Motte's study of opium in a newspaper article from 1922, indicating that he at least maintained respect for her efforts, and it is hard to believe that the two would not have crossed paths in the course of their common crusade against opium, but if they did there are no letters documenting the content and extent of their contact. In 1919, after her interview with Winslow, she typed up a report to explain how she and Chadbourne met Das and the nature of their relationship in an effort to explain away the behavior that the American and British authorities found suspect. She, too, described meeting him on the *Tenyo Maru* on the way to Japan and the lectures he gave on deck, which she found "frank and free."[166] He also lectured on the "opium traffic as an example of European methods of reducing a conquered country to docility,"[167] a topic that clearly resonated with her; she undoubtedly had thought about the effects of opium as present in the medications administered to her patients during the war and in Baltimore, but presumably Das' connecting of opium to politics and colonialism was an awakening for her. Interestingly, her report devoted only this one line to the topic despite the fact that it had begun to consume her life and would do so for more than a dozen years.

Much of the report provides explanations for various actions that the British authorities had interpreted as signaling La Motte and Chadbourne's intention to actively support Das' anti-British revolutionary views. For example, she describes meeting with him in Tokyo and Shanghai, "often in the lobby of the hotel," where they were willing to meet in public because they were "Not … in the slightest degree conscious of his being a suspicious character," thus they "talked to him as freely and openly, in public places, as heart could wish."[168] These meetings had damaging consequences: La Motte reported that in March 1918, "a friend told us what she considered a 'joke' on us," which her friend "had hesitated to tell us, as she thought it so impertinent, but she said, it was too funny to keep to herself any longer."[169] The gist was that she was warned by "a gentleman" to "Have nothing to do with those two ladies. They are dangerous characters."[170] His source of information was "a British Secret Service man who told every body in the bar, 'Have nothing to do with those two ladies–they are fomenting a revolution in India.' "[171] Belatedly learning that their innocent talks with Das had been so misconstrued as to label them enemies of the British, La Motte reflected on other meetings with him that had probably been assigned other nefarious intentions. She describes interviewing him because she "was very anxious to write the story of Das' early life" so met with him frequently "in the lobby of the Imperial Hotel, Tokyo, with pad and pencil … I suppose that looked awful, but being unconscious of fomenting a revolution, that's what I did."[172] On another occasion, they wanted to make curry so they went to the home of some "Hindu friends" of Das where "they cooked us all kinds of Indian dishes."[173] All of these visits were in fact construed by the British to be evidence of their potential involvement in incriminating activities, for they could not understand their communication with Das and other Hindus as marked by anything other than malicious intent.

Particularly damning were the financial links between them. In his report of June 6, 1917, Agent S. reported that La Motte and Chadbourne had given Das money as they were departing Tokyo, another action that implicated them with Das' political activities, yet La Motte defends what they did by explaining that Chadbourne had purchased some cups from "a Chinese gentleman," and since she had not had the opportunity to pay him back, they, at the very last minute "as the last rope was being cast off from the dock," gave Das the money and asked him to pay the man back.[174] La Motte confesses that it must have looked suspect and that "Doubtless every British Secret Service man on the dock saw me handing money to Das," yet she queried, "Dont [*sic*] you think if I had been really financing a revolution I would have been a little less brazen about it?"[175]

She also addresses the issue of paying Das' bail, something that they did not see as a political act but as compensation to Das for their own advice. She explains that because they fully believed in his innocence and in his assertion that he "deplored violence" in favor of education as a means of advocating for Indian independence, she had encouraged him to travel to the United States to focus on "mastering the English language" so "he would then be equipped when the war ended, to go on with his educational work."[176] As her intercepted letter of August 17, 1917 shows, she also wanted him to come to defend himself and clear his name. Believing in his innocence and feeling guilty, they "bailed him out" and "got him a lawyer" because they "felt responsible for his coming to this country" and "felt we must help him."[177] Although La Motte presents their motivations as emerging from a sense of personal indebtedness, her report makes clear that she was sympathetic to the larger implications of his goals and situation when she observed that because he was "an American citizen (naturalized), and having committed no act for which the British could ask the U.S.A. to hand him over to them, he was subject to an amazing sort of persecution."[178] Her sense of outrage at the way a foreign government could harass an American citizen even when he had not broken any laws was compounded by her view of the legitimacy of attempting to establish an independent India. As she says in a typically trenchant comment, "You can see why they [British authorities] wanted him. There was a lot of talk in those days about the tragedy of Belgium, and a person who goes about wanting to un-Belgium other parts of the works is persona non grata."[179] La Motte ultimately distanced herself from Das in this report, but she shared his sense of the injustice of Britain's dominating India while denouncing Germany for its conquests in Europe.

La Motte processed the experience of being subject to surveillance in an unpublished story, "The Spy." In it, she imagines a room filled with workers who are divided into groups according to their expertise: some could read "various languages," others focused on "trade letters" or "banking letters," and there are even some allocated to a room where "the privileged mail was examined, those letters supposed to be exempt from all censorship."[180] Her narrator, however, eschews those areas to focus on "the many tables where the ordinary social letters were deposited."[181] The narrator then introduces a cast of readers, workers like Katharine, who "enjoyed it–after the first day" when she had to overcome the "old conventions" and "good breeding" to steel herself to open mail belonging to other people.[182]

Her colleague next to her scans the letters, searching for "good little tips on the market," and another stores away the names of people who had written "very foolish, indiscreet letters," which he plans to use later when "there might be troubled times, without employment, when such items would come in handy."[183] In their midst sits "a spy," "audacious, dangerous," whom the others denounce "indignant[ly]" once she is found out.[184] Having pointed out the hypocrisy of the workers' actions, the narrator does not share their outrage and sarcastically highlights "their different standards and degrees of honor" and comments that "war is a very undermining business, take it from whatever angle. It exacts a price."[185] The price, the story makes clear, is the loss of morals and standards the workers experience even as they are purportedly working on behalf of a higher cause: their nation. Ironically, it is only the spy who has truly pure motives and is dedicated to serving the greater good instead of herself.

La Motte wrote the story in the fall of 1919 when she was at Yama Farms, one of the locations she visited frequently in the summers of 1918–1920. She also made trips to other Ulster County, NY, locations such as Ladleton, NY, where she was thirty miles from the train, fourteen miles from the nearest telephone, several miles from a post office, and with no access to a telegraph–a spot she said she "loved" and where she learned to "run a Ford,"[186] the beginning of her love of driving that would last the rest of her life–and to Woodstock at the invitation of friends.[187] Yama Farms, however, appears to have been a favorite haunt. Located near Wawarsing, NY, it was an unusual inn built by Frank Seaman, who made a fortune in advertising, and his wife, Olive Brown Sarre, with Japanese-style buildings and gardens.[188] It was frequented by barons of industry such as Thomas Edison, Henry Ford, and Harvey Firestone, and served as a gathering spot for intellectuals and artists.[189]

La Motte's time in New York, during which she was writing and waiting for permission to obtain a new passport, was also marked by using her nursing skills–for the first time since she left the hospital in Belgium in June 1916–at an influenza hospital in October 1918.[190] She subsequently contracted influenza but was fortunate enough to recover after a month of convalescence.[191] She had a support network of friends in the city, one that was probably supplemented by the intellectual and artistic milieu of the women of the Heterodoxy–a club that began meeting in 1912 in Greenwich Village.[192] The conditions for membership were loose: two dollars a year and having an "unorthodox" point of view.[193] The group included artists, journalists, lawyers, and writers, many of them with progressive views that they could safely share and debate while exploring topics such as "pacifism, birth control, the Russian Revolution … health issues, infant mortality, anarchism … education of women, Black civil rights, disabled women, the Irish independence movement, free love, psychology, and so much more."[194] Given the practice of not publicizing or sharing attendance at meetings or the topics under discussion, there are no records to verify when La Motte joined this group, but in 1920 members presented their founder, Marie Jenney Howe,[195] with an album of photographs and inscriptions. La Motte's is to be found a little more than halfway through, her inscription reading, "As to message–just greetings to all my dear Heterodoxy friends and lets [*sic*] always keep step with the March of Time."[196] On a list of members found by scholar Patricia McClelland Miller in the papers of Helen Hull, La Motte's address is identified as "China," thus revealing that she had joined Heterodoxy at least by summer 1916, when she left for her travels in Asia.[197]

Who introduced her to the group is unknown, but she would have been thrilled to be a member of the same club as Charlotte Perkins Gilman, a writer she admired and read.[198] It may have been Inez Haynes Gillmore Irwin, in whose papers the Howe album ended up, who invited her to attend meetings. Irwin's unpublished diary from 1916 describes meeting "Mrs. Chadbourne … and a Miss Ellen La Motte" through friends while on a trip to Paris.[199] Irwin offers a rare first impression of both women: she describes Chadbourne as being "very beautiful … in a slightly-faded, etiolated way. She is of what is called 'an uncertain age' and she has a low, rather monotonous voice. She wore an extraordinary necklace of gold suspending a huge hexagonal, translucent green stone. In her smart Cossack-like, black-furred cap was another huge, hexagonal translucent green stone. She told me they were East Indian emeralds–flawed; she has six of them."[200] In contrast to this opulence, she describes La Motte as "dark, tall, big, simply dressed in the plainest of suits, very vigorous in her speech and in her movements."[201] Irwin summarizes their conversation: La Motte recounted being under bombardment in Dunkirk and used

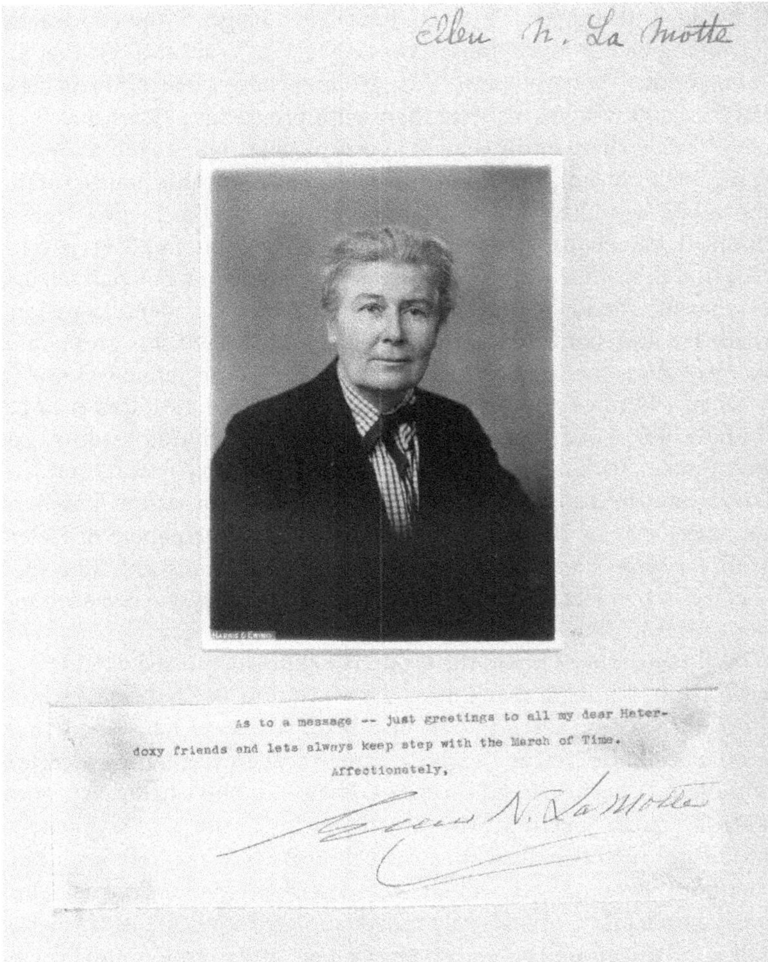

Figure 9 Portrait of La Motte from the "Heterodoxy to Marie" scrapbook of photographs and appreciations from members of the Heterodoxy club to Marie Jenney Howe [1920]

language similar to that in her article, "Under Shell-Fire at Dunkirk." Irwin recorded that La Motte recounted, "'I never was in a position,' she said, 'when any previous experience or any previous training was of so little use,'"[202] an echo of her observation in her article that "there was not one intellectual faculty I could call upon. There was nothing in past experience, nothing of will-power, of judgment, of intuition, that could serve me."[203]

Irwin met them several months later "in a beautiful apartment, exquisitely furnished." She gushes, "I can't enumerate all the beautiful things I saw but they included furniture of the periods of the various Louises (what is the plural of Louis?); furniture in Chinese Chippendale; Gaugins [*sic*]; Cezannes [*sic*]; one beautiful, big old chest, filled only with marvelous stuffs … jewelry …."[204] She describes, "a filet, made with small leaves of gold, berries of agate and lapis dew drops of diamonds; a chain suspending a great oval pendant and set with huge cabochon stones, quite indescribable, made by a woman artist. And to go with it, a comb, very delicate, of silver, with tiny mistletoe leaves in green enamel and mistletoe berries of pearls … I have never seen such a collection."[205] She undoubtedly saw pieces by Florence Koehler, a jeweler who worked in Chicago and with whom Chadbourne was friends.[206] Chadbourne commissioned Koehler to make various pieces for her that she later donated to the Metropolitan Museum of Art.[207] She was also shown a guest room, "very elaborate and magnificent" with "a beautiful, painted, wooden bed which they bought in Spain for ten francs" and "a row of quaint, white-wigged women portraits, painted on glass, which they purchased in Spain and carried all the way to France in their hands."[208] Mrs. Chadbourne's bedroom was a stark contrast to the luxury of the rest of the house, consisting of nothing but a bed and "a shrine with a crucifix."[209] Irwin saw them again at a later date the day before La Motte's third trip to *L'Hôpital Chirurgical Mobile No. 1*. She describes having a "delicious meal and a dull talk with an old dope who has the correct information on nothing and the wrong ideas about everything. However the conversation wakes up when there drop in two ambulanciers … and a nurse, who has been serving nine months in a hospital."[210] Apparently, Irwin preferred their conversation about "plugging up appendicitis incisions by pouring the wound as full of ether as it will hold," a welcome change of pace from that of the "old dope."[211] It is reasonable to assume that Irwin, after these encounters in Paris, may have subsequently invited La Motte to join a Heterodoxy meeting once she moved back to the United States; La Motte would have made a logical addition given her professional background and extensive experience as a speaker and writer. She would have relished engaging in debates with other intelligent women and profited from testing her own ideas in energetic conversations with them as she continued work in the anti-opium campaign.

Her ideas regarding the dangers of opium received further endorsement when she signed a contract for her fifth book, *The Opium Monopoly*, with Macmillan in October of 1919. The book, published in January 1920, offers a brief introduction to how she became interested in the opium trade–through meeting Das–and why the opium monopoly is such a difficult problem to solve: governments generate revenue through "the sale of opium, through excise taxes upon opium, and through license fees paid by the keepers of opium shops and divans."[212] Given this lucrative business, which she reveals through study of "official blue books and government reports, issued by the British Government," there is little motivation for these governments to abandon their parts in the monopoly.[213] She marvels that these truths are so easily available in these official documents, yet the American people know very little of the extent of the opium trade. In order to make this subject relevant to her primary reading audience in the United States, she points out that "The menace of opium is now threatening America ... Little by little, surreptitiously, this drug has been creeping in over our borders, and today many thousands of our young men and young women are drug addicts, habituated to the use of one of the opium derivatives, morphia or heroin."[214] She supports her claim by discussing what she saw during the "first week of the opening of the Health Department Clinic for Drug Addicts in New York City" when she took "the histories of these pitiful, abject wrecks of men and women who swarmed to the clinic in hundreds, seeking supplies of the drug which they could not obtain elsewhere."[215] The only way to prevent the devastating consequences of addiction, affecting the young in particular, is to clamp down on "over-production, the sole object of which is to create drug victims."[216] She states that the only way forward with accomplishing such a goal is to create "a moral sentiment" in the populations of both England and the United States to encourage the people to join together in articulating a demand the stop overproduction.

The goals are lofty and prescient given the degree to which drug addiction would plague the United States in the twentieth and twenty-first centuries, yet the book itself consists primarily of staid government reports, which only the most engaged readers could find stimulating. Once she describes, using a long selection from Samuel Merwin's 1908 book, *Drugging a Nation*, how the British government serves as "the source of supply" for opium and finances the growing of opium in India, which is then sold at monthly auctions; she squarely assigns responsibility to the British for overproducing opium that is subsequently "turned loose upon the world, to bring destruction and ruin to the human race."[217] Drawing heavily on official documents she charts how the monopoly functions by examining the role in it of various countries, primarily in Asia and the Middle East.

In her analysis, she returns to how race plays into policies on opium consumption after musing about an article she had read regarding the arrest of a number of Chinese nationals in an opium den in England. She comments that it must have been confusing

> [t]o come from a part of the British Empire where opium smoking is freely encouraged, to Great Britain itself where such practices are not tolerated. He [the arrested Chinese citizen] must ask himself, why it is that the white race is so sedulously protected from such vices, while the subject races are so eagerly encouraged … Subject races, dependents, who have no vote, no share in the government and who are powerless to protect themselves–fair game for exploitation. Is this double-dealing what we mean when we speak of "our responsibility to backward nations," or of "the sacred trust of civilization," or still again when we refer to "the White Man's burden?"[218]

She returns to these arguments in the conclusion, when she takes apart the claim that opium "is not harmful–if taken in moderation."[219] If it is as safe as its defenders assert, it is odd that "those European countries which derive much profit through the sale of opium to their subject races, seem to have an aversion to introducing it to their people at home."[220]

These arguments are treated anew in *The Ethics of Opium*, the contract for which she signed in New York in November of 1923; by February 1924 the book was in circulation. It continues the familiar arguments made in *The Opium Monopoly* with a particular focus on the dangers of overproduction. Once again, she tries to interest the American reader by highlighting the dangers the trade, impossibly distant from the point of view of most Americans, posed to the welfare of the citizens of the United States. This overproduction, she points out, results in "overflow … that must necessarily filter back into Europe and America."[221] Making her audience see the danger of that overflow and its menace to the young, "the fresh, the unspoiled," given that those under twenty are most likely to become addicted to drugs, is an important part of the rhetorical appeal she makes in the text.[222] However, like her previous book, it would most likely draw in readers already heavily invested in the topic given its incorporation of facts and figures taken from official government documents and its uninspired organization by country, covering a number of places mentioned in *The Opium Monopoly*. It is a long read at 205 pages, and it is difficult to imagine that many readers, except for existing students of the topic, would endeavor to read it cover to cover.

Perhaps more effective in piquing the interest of the public was the series of articles she published about opium in journals and magazines, including the *Atlantic Monthly*, the *Nation*, *Harper's Magazine*, the *New Freeman*, the *American Journal of Nursing*, and the *Trained Nurse and Hospital Review*, between 1922 and 1934. These articles make many of the same points about the dangers of overproduction, the abuse of colonized people as a result of the opium trade, and the subsequent threat to Americans at risk of becoming addicts that are made in her book-length studies of opium. However, most of the articles are short, around two to three pages long, and focused on discrete points that the average readers of these magazines could quickly digest. La Motte collected much of the material for these pieces on her frequent trips to Geneva, headquarters of the League of Nations. As of fall 1920, she and Chadbourne had set off for Europe, first landing in Paris and then traveling to London, where they decided to go so that they could truly engage in their "opium campaign … right [at] headquarters, and do [their] fighting on the spot."[223] They spent the next twelve years based in London but frequently visiting Geneva to attend meetings of the Opium Committee of the League of Nations, an organization in which she did not believe,[224] after which La Motte would report back via these brief pieces in an effort to keep the pressure on the nations involved in these negotiations to stamp out overproduction and the illicit sale of opium.

During this period, she was highly invested, indeed consumed, by the topic of opium and the injustices she saw perpetuated by its production and sale. Her work was her primary focus, and she took pride in her ability to rattle those defending the drug.[225] She did, however, return to short fiction as a mechanism for exploring the hypocrisies of opium policies and the conflict between East and West in her seventh and last book, *Snuffs and Butters*. She signed the contract with Century in May 1924; the book was published in the spring of 1925 and included three stories that had appeared as early as 1919 and 1920 in *Century Magazine*. The collection received fewer reviews that her previous works though they tended to be complimentary; one in the *New York Times* critiqued the first story in the collection, "Snuffs and Butters," in which a Chinese citizen is arrested for innocently taking opium into England to help his sick son–he does not realize the substance, legally for sale in his homeland, is banned in Britain–for having a "crusading spirit'; however, the reviewer credited others, for example those dealing with love, as being, "poignant and adroitly treat[ing]" their subject.[226]

La Motte also continued to evolve personally; turning fifty in 1923, she continued to challenge herself through work, travel, and writing about topics other than opium. One story, written in the same year, although she waited until 1930 to send it to *Harper's*, who rejected it, returned to her concern about gender and social justice. "Murderers Who Escape" recounts the rape and subsequent death of a ten-year-old girl whose father kills his daughter's rapist out of a belief that the law would do nothing to her killer. Justice, however, is swiftly brought to bear against the father and he is sentenced to life in prison. He eventually goes insane in prison to "escape" the horror of incarceration; the story suggests that the father, the one who experienced the grievous loss of his daughter, has suffered more punishment than the man who raped and killed his child. Between 1926 and 1929, La Motte continued to work on her fiction and wrote a series of stories, *Our Street: Stories and Sketches of London*, that was never published except for two pieces, "A Desert Owl" and "Hidden Treasure," which appeared in the *Atlantic Monthly* in January 1927 and August 1928. The collection focuses on a small cast of characters who live in formerly grand houses that have fallen into disrepair, like many of their inhabitants, who once had more money or social status. They are primarily middle-aged women who struggle with loneliness as they try to hold on to their former dignity. In sharp contrast to these meek and reserved women, the unpublished story "The Psychology of Bobbing," which she submitted to the *Atlantic Monthly* and *Century Magazine* and sent to Mencken asking him to consider it for *American Mercury*,[227] explores from the first-person perspective of "Ellen," who rejoices in the freedom of cutting her hair, hair, she says, "that kept me back, from expanding ... that stood for inhibitions, and timidities, and conventions, and shynesses and spiritual shackles of all kinds."[228] After bragging to her friends and fishing for compliments on her bold new hairdo, she is sagely advised by a lawyer friend, "Elinor,"[229] to go home and write down her exultation, "This amazing exhilaration. A return to youth perhaps. A proof, somehow, that your mind is still young enough, still flexible enough to take in a new idea," before the feeling fades.[230]

Testing her flexibility was something she continued to do in the 1920s: in February 1926 she went on a trip on the Nile and spent approximately six weeks traveling from Cairo to Wadi Halfa, just across the border in Sudan. On one houseboat, the *Fostat*, were members of the Crane family[231] and on the other, the *Scarab*, a smaller and slower boat, La Motte, Emily Chadbourne, D. M. Brodie, Matthew Stewart Prichard, Henri de Beaumont, and Thomas Whittemore.[232] She kept a daily diary of this trip to record her impressions of the surrounding environment and antiquities they visited under the tutelage of Whittemore, who was particularly interested in seeing Coptic churches. In between noting the names of temples, she made observations regarding the development of the Egyptians, towards whom she had mixed views: at times she judged them for the poverty in which some lived and at others she recognized that after fifty years of occupation by the British, any "benefit has come to the prople [*sic*] ... as a side issue, a by-product."[233]

While on the trip, she wrote a short story, "The Assuan Dam," about Aziz, a Nubian, who loses his strip of rich farmland alongside the Nile when it is flooded when the Aswan Low Dam was built, revealing deep empathy for those displaced by this modern feat of engineering that offered little benefit to those whose livelihoods were disrupted by

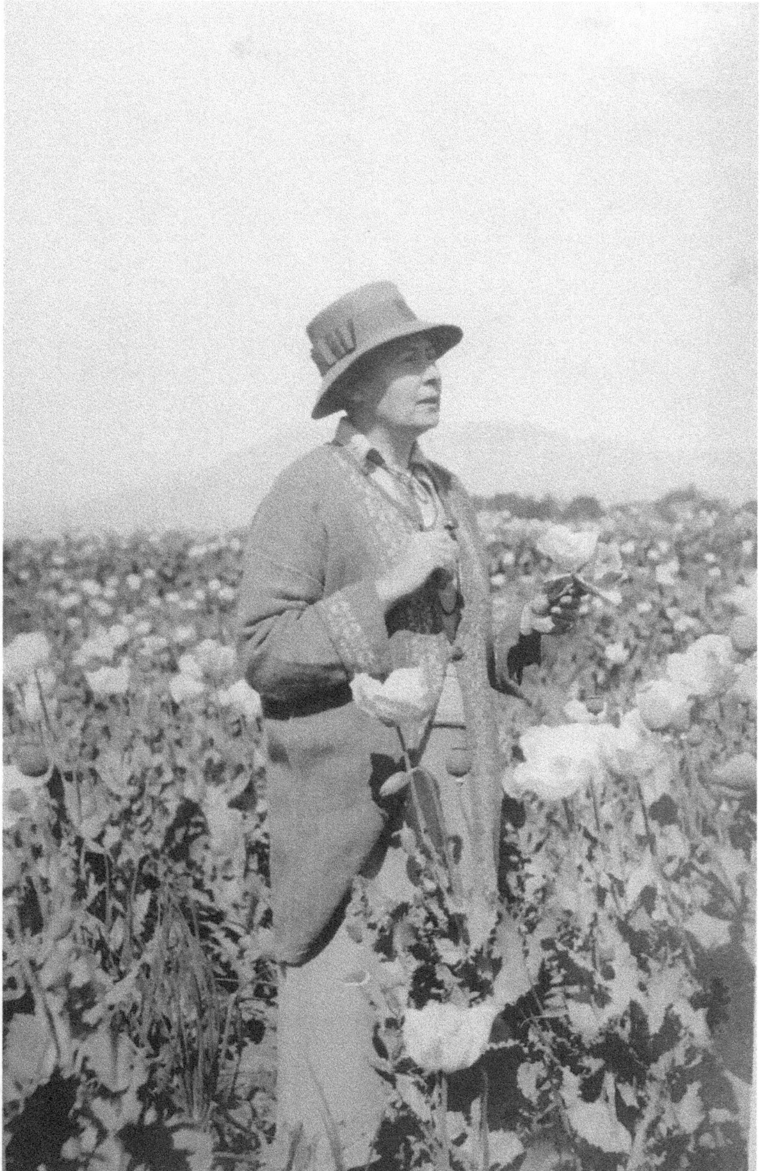

Figure 10 La Motte, Luxor, Egypt, 1926

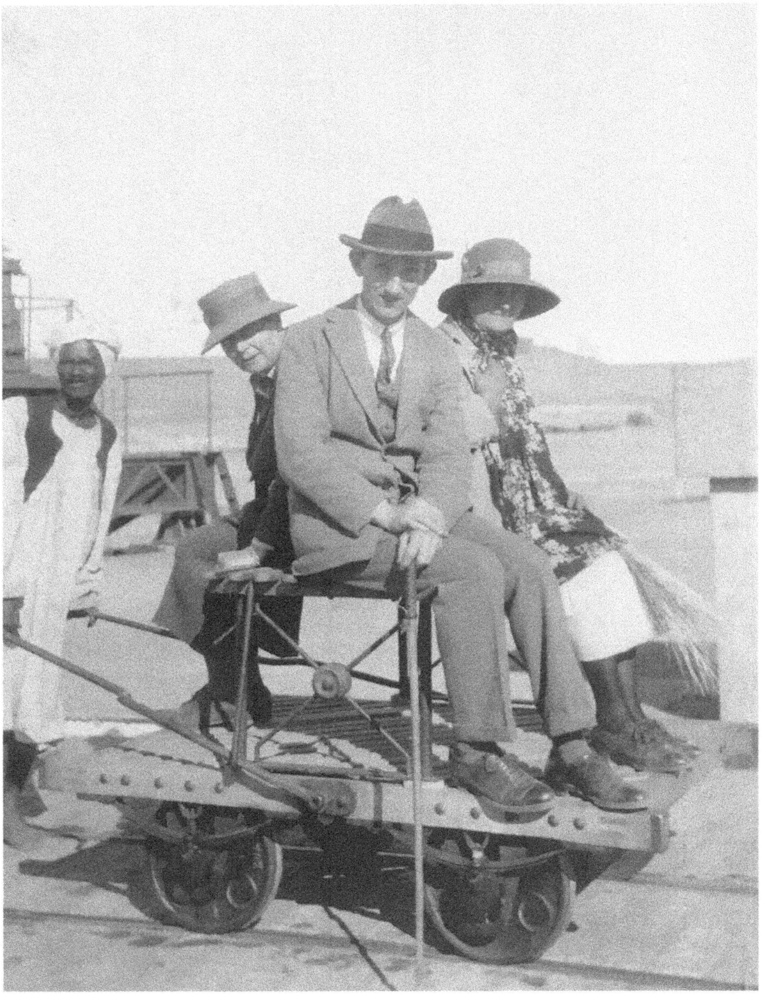

Figure 11 La Motte and friends, Assuan Dam, Egypt, 1926

its construction. The trip offered La Motte the opportunity to return to her opium preoccupation when she tried to buy some in Esna and visited several opium fields, where she had her photograph taken, something, Chadbourne told Stein, that made La Motte "delighted with herself."[234]

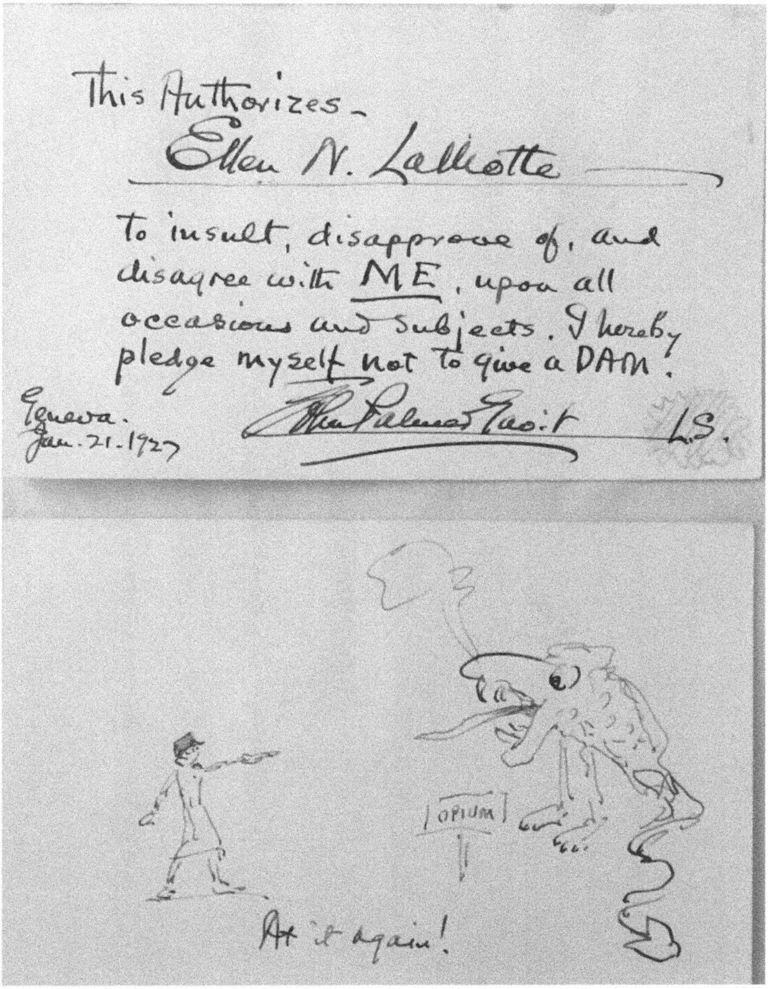

Figure 12 Sketch given to La Motte by John Palmer Gavit, 1927

Soon after their return from Egypt, Chadbourne emptied her Paris apartment, gave great quantities of artworks to the Art Institute of Chicago,[235] and made 2000 Massachusetts Avenue in Washington, DC her home base. The two women continued to travel a great deal separately, with La Motte moving apartments

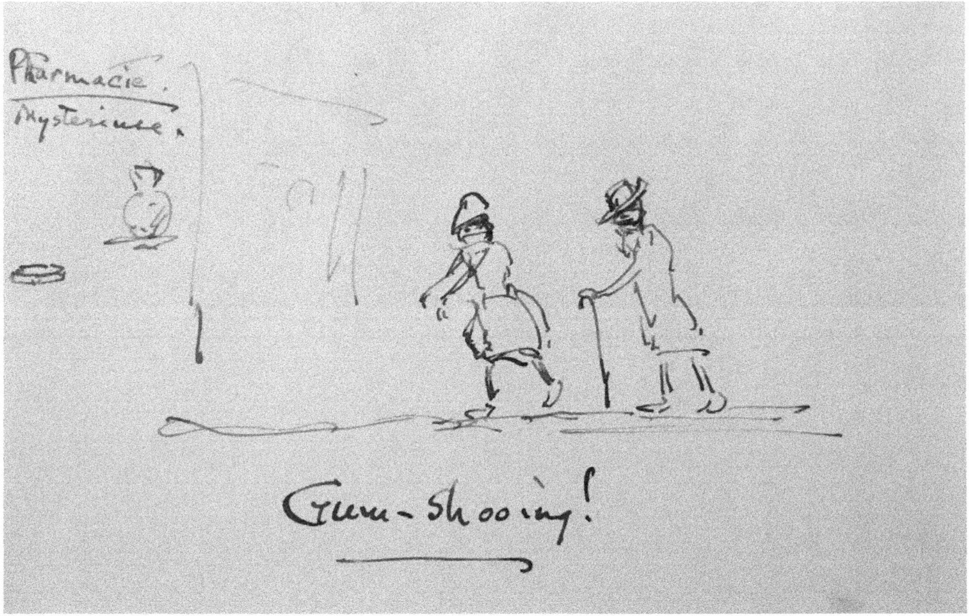

Figure 13 Sketch given to La Motte by John Palmer Gavit, 1927

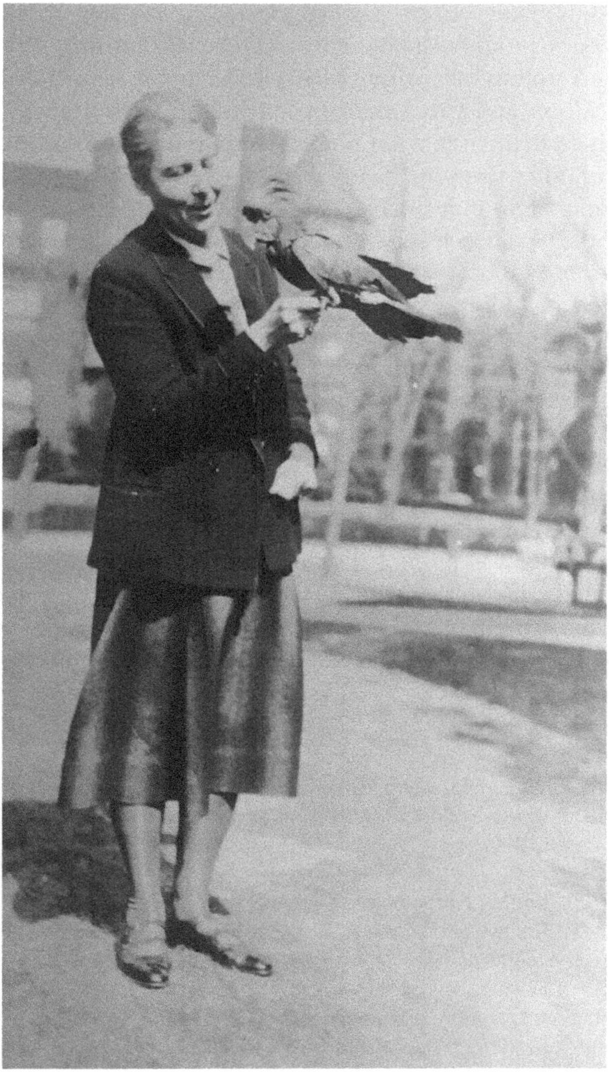

Figure 14 Portrait of La Motte with cockatoo

in London, from where she concentrated on her writing and continued making frequent visits to Geneva, "fanning" the flames in the anti-opium campaign.[236] Despite having three articles placed in the *Nation* and the *American Journal of Nursing* in 1929, she complained to Stein that her finances and writing were at the lowest ebb[237]–a far cry from the heady days of a year earlier when she was bragging to Stein that she had earned $600.

Over the next two years she published two anti-opium pieces in the *New Freeman* and several short stories and travel pieces in *Harper's* and the *Nation*, including a racist account of traveling to Ethiopia to watch the coronation of Haile Selassie. These, however, would be among her last published works. Although two short pieces related to opium were published by the *Nation* in 1932 and 1934, interest in the topic was on the wane, given the global economic depression preoccupying much of the world and the building threat of another major worldwide conflict. By November 1931, La Motte announced to her cousin that she was returning permanently to the United States.[238] After more than a decade of hopping between London, Paris, Geneva, and the United States, La Motte, living in more straitened circumstances and nearing her sixtieth birthday, settled into the place, Washington, DC, that would shape and redefine the last decades of her life.

Notes

1 "Mostly about People," *News Journal* (Wilmington, DE) (August 2, 1916), p. 9.
2 "Former Nurse is Seeking Respite from War's Roar," *San Francisco Chronicle* (August 24, 1916), p. 6.
3 *Ibid.*
4 GSABTP, "Emily Chadbourne to Gertrude Stein," July 4, 1915.
5 GSABTP, "Emily Chadbourne to Gertrude Stein," December 19, 1915.
6 Gertrude Stein, *The Autobiography of Alice B. Toklas* (New York: Vintage, 1990), p. 158.
7 See Chapter 3 for more discussion of this comment.
8 Private Collection, "Ellen N. La Motte to Ellen Newbold La Motte," May 31, 1916.
9 Jane Conway, *A Woman of Two Wars: The Life of Mary Borden* (London: Munday, 2010), p. 50.
10 La Motte, according to the first edition of *The Backwash of War*, wrote "The Interval' in Paris on May 9, 1916 and "Locomotor Ataxia" on June 18, 1916;

see Ellen N. La Motte, *The Backwash of War* (New York: G. P. Putnam's Sons, 1916), pp. 92 and 140. The postcard to her mother places her at the hospital on May 31, 1916, suggesting she spent another three or four weeks there in the interval between stories.

11 She visited Boston and Wilmington, according to "Mostly about People," p. 9, before departing on her "tour around the world."

12 Ellen N. Lamotte, "*The Backwash of War*, Picture of Hell," *Evening Sun* (September 30, 1916), p. 6.

13 Burleson to Postmasters of the First, Second, and Third Classes, cited in D. Johnson, "Wilson, Burleson, and Censorship in the First World War," *Journal of Southern History* 28:1 (February 1962), p. 48.

14 NARA, Records of the Office of the Solicitor, Post Office Department, "Elmer McBroom to Solicitor," August 20, 1917.

15 NARA, Records of the Office of the Solicitor, Post Office Department, "J. J. Southerland, Acting Solicitor, to Elmer McBroom," August 29, 1917.

16 NARA, Records of the Office of the Solicitor, Post Office Department, "Robert A. Bowen to William H. Lamar," May 27, 1918.

17 *Ibid.*

18 *Ibid.*

19 *Ibid.*

20 William J. Maxwell, *F. B. Eyes: How J. Edgar Hoover's Ghostreaders Framed African American Literature* (Princeton, NJ: Princeton University Press, 2015), p. 194.

21 *Ibid.*

22 Robert Adger Bowen, "The Alien Problem," *Greenville News* (August 15, 1937), p. 6.

23 See Maxwell for a discussion of how this office and the FBI monitored the writings and activities of African American artists and intellectuals.

24 NARA, Records of the Office of the Solicitor, Post Office Department, "Memo for the Solicitor," July 26, 1918.

25 NARA, Records of the Office of the Solicitor, Post Office Department, "Lamar to Bowen," July 26, 1918.

26 See Peter Conolly-Smith, "'Reading between the Lines': The Bureau of Investigation, the United States Post Office, and Domestic Surveillance during World War I," *Social Justice* 36:1 (2009), pp. 7–24, for a discussion of the connections between the Department of Justice and the Post Office following the declaration of war and the passing of the Espionage and Trading with the Enemy Acts of 1917. See also Johnson, "Wilson, Burleson, and Censorship."

27 Conolly-Smith, "'Reading between the Lines,'" p. 7.

28 NARA, Records of the Office of the Solicitor, Post Office Department, "Ellen N. La Motte to Albert S. Burleson," December 7, 1918.

29 NARA, Records of the Office of the Solicitor, Post Office Department, "Solicitor to Ellen N. La Motte," December 30, 1917.
30 Johnson, "Wilson, Burleson, and Censorship," p. 57.
31 See Chapter 4 for a discussion of the *Masses*' endorsement of La Motte's book and naming of her as a kind of honorary contributing editor.
32 See Chapter 4 for a discussion of the reaction by some of her colleagues in Borden Turner's hospital to the contents of her book.
33 Chadbourne sent Toklas a postcard from Hawaii in early September; see GSABTP, "Chadbourne to Toklas," September 1, 1916; and La Motte sent Stein a postcard from Garden of the Gods in Colorado, although she mailed it from the boat, en route to Japan, one day out of Yokohama; see GSABTP, "La Motte to Stein," September 10, 1916.
34 Ellen N. La Motte, *Peking Dust* (New York: Century Company, 1919), p. 4.
35 *Ibid.*, p. 83. La Motte describes their trip to Cambodia in Ellen N. La Motte, "The Ruins of Angkor," *Harper's Magazine* (February 1920), pp. 364–378.
36 Taraknath Das, *The Free Hindusthan*, April 1908, p. 1.
37 Ronald Spector, "The Vermont Education of Taraknath Das: An Episode in British-American-Indian Relations," *Proceedings of the Vermont Historical Society* 48:2 (Spring 1980), p. 91.
38 *Ibid.*, p. 93.
39 *Ibid.*, p. 94.
40 Ellen N. La Motte, *The Opium Monopoly* (New York: Macmillan, 1920), pp. ix–x.
41 *Ibid.*, p. x.
42 *Ibid.*
43 Tapan K. Mukherjee, *Taraknath Das: Life and Letters of a Revolutionary in Exile* (Calcutta: National Council of Education, 1998), p. 105.
44 *Ibid.*
45 Private Collection, Ellen N. La Motte, *Drafts of Unfinished Stories and Sketches, 1911–1919* (hereafter *Drafts*), "Cripples."
46 "Fifth American Victim of Shell," *New York Times* (April 4, 1018), p. 13.
47 La Motte, *Drafts*, "To Emma G. Mullen."
48 "The Reasons for 'Peking Dust,'" *Des Moines Register* (April 13, 1919), p. 37.
49 *Ibid.*
50 La Motte, *Peking Dust*, p. 3.
51 *Ibid.*, p. 24
52 *Ibid.*, p. 25.
53 *Ibid.*, pp. 28–29.
54 La Motte, *The Backwash of War*, p. vi.
55 *Ibid.*
56 La Motte, *Peking Dust*, pp. 27, 28.
57 *Ibid.*, p. 75.
58 *Ibid.*, p. 50.

59 *Ibid.*
60 *Ibid.*, p. 51.
61 *Ibid.*, p. 63.
62 *Ibid.*, p. 127.
63 *Ibid.*, p. 128.
64 *Ibid.*, p. 129.
65 *Ibid.*, p. 131.
66 *Ibid.*, p. 201.
67 *Ibid.*, p. 197.
68 *Ibid.*
69 *Ibid.*, p. 229.
70 *Ibid.*, p. 230.
71 *Ibid.*
72 *Ibid.*
73 Mencken Papers (hereafter MP), Manuscripts and Archives Division, The New York Public Library, "Ellen N. La Motte to H. L. Mencken," August 5, 1918.
74 "Orient Made Grim," *New York Tribune* (May 24, 1919), p. 11.
75 "Masculine Vigor in Miss La Motte's Tales," *Evening Sun* (June 21, 1919), p. 6.
76 Ellen N. La Motte, "The Yellow Streak," in *Civilization: Tales of the Orient* (New York: George H. Doran, 1919), p. 11.
77 *Ibid.*, p. 12.
78 *Ibid.*, p. 13.
79 *Ibid.*, p. 16.
80 *Ibid.*
81 *Ibid.*, pp. 18–19.
82 *Ibid.*, p. 19.
83 *Ibid.*, p. 19, 20.
84 *Ibid.*, p. 20.
85 *Ibid.*, p. 21.
86 *Ibid.*
87 *Ibid.*, p. 23.
88 *Ibid.*, p. 26
89 *Ibid.*, p. 28.
90 *Ibid.*, p. 29.
91 *Ibid.*
92 La Motte, "On the Heights," in *Civilization: Tales of the Orient*, p. 33.
93 *Ibid.*, p. 39.
94 *Ibid.*, p. 40.
95 *Ibid.*, p. 44–45.
96 *Ibid.*, p. 53.
97 *Ibid.*, p. 55.
98 *Ibid.*, p. 61.

99 La Motte, "Homesick," in *Civilization: Tales of the Orient*, pp. 68, 69.
100 *Ibid.*
101 La Motte, "Prisoners," in *Civilization: Tales of the Orient*, p. 142.
102 *Ibid.*, p. 143.
103 *Ibid.*, pp. 156.
104 *Ibid.*, pp. 158.
105 *Ibid.*, pp. 160.
106 *Ibid.*
107 *Ibid.*, p. 164.
108 *Ibid.*, p. 167.
109 *Ibid.*, p. 171.
110 La Motte, "Civilization," in *Civilization: Tales of the Orient*, pp. 105–106.
111 *Ibid.*, p. 106.
112 *Ibid.*, p. 107.
113 *Ibid.*, p. 113.
114 *Ibid.*, p. 117.
115 La Motte, "Cholera," in *Civilization: Tales of the Orient*, p. 241.
116 La Motte, *Peking Dust*, p. 56.
117 *Ibid.*, p. 57.
118 La Motte, "Under a Wineglass," in *Civilization: Tales of the Orient*, p. 224.
119 *Ibid.*
120 *Ibid.*, p. 219.
121 *Ibid.*, p. 226.
122 *Ibid.*, p. 228.
123 *Ibid.*, p. 231.
124 *Ibid.*, p. 227.
125 See the Introduction and Chapter 3 for discussion of La Motte and Chadbourne's relationship.
126 La Motte, "Canterbury Chimes," in *Civilization: Tales of the Orient*, p. 177.
127 *Ibid.*, p. 194.
128 *Ibid.*, p. 196.
129 *Ibid.*, p. 190.
130 She told her cousin, Alfred I. du Pont, that he no longer needed to send her a stipend since "my little writings bring me in enough to get along on." See AID, "Ellen N. La Motte to Alfred I. du Pont," May 3, 1918.
131 AID, "Ellen N. La Motte to Alfred I. du Pont," June 30, 1918.
132 AID, "Alfred I. du Pont to Ellen N. La Motte," February 8, 1918.
133 *Ibid.*
134 NARA, Investigative Reports of the Bureau of Investigation 1908–1922, Old German Files, 1909–1921, "Chief to Charles DeWoody," May 4, 1918.
135 NARA, Investigative Reports of the Bureau of Investigation 1908–1922, Old German Files, 1909–1921, "Charles DeWoody to A. Bruce Bielaski," May 9, 1918.

136 *Ibid.*
137 NARA, Record Group 60: Records of the Department of Justice, "L. Lanier Winslow to John Lord O'Brian," May 16, 1919.
138 *Ibid.*
139 *Ibid.*
140 *Ibid.*
141 *Ibid.*
142 NARA, Investigative Reports of the Bureau of Investigation 1908–1922, Old German Files, 1909–1921, "Charles DeWoody to A. Bruce Bielaski," May 9, 1918.
143 The National Archives, Kew (hereafter TNA), Foreign Office, FO 115/2236, "Thomas Hohler to Leland Harrison," September 11, 1917.
144 TNA, Foreign Office, FO 115/2235, "C. J. Davidson to Conyngham Greene," May 29, 1917.
145 TNA, Foreign Office, FO 115/2235, "Conyngham Greene to Arthur Balfour," June 1, 1917.
146 TNA, Foreign Office, FO 115/2235, "Conyngham Greene to Arthur Balfour," June 6, 1917.
147 *Ibid.*
148 TNA, Foreign Office, FO 115/2235, "Report by Agent S.," June 6, 1917.
149 *Ibid.*
150 TNA, Foreign Office, FO 115/2235, "Report by Agent P.," June 10, 1917.
151 TNA, Foreign Office, FO 115/2235, "Conyngham Greene to Arthur Balfour," June 12, 1917.
152 See Chapter 4 for a discussion of *Backwash* and the immediate reaction to it.
153 TNA, Foreign Office, FO 115/2235, "Conyngham Greene to Arthur Balfour," June 12, 1917.
154 TNA, Foreign Office, FO 115/2236, "Richard Gottheil to 'Your Excellency,'" August 13, 1917.
155 TNA, Foreign Office, FO 115/2236, "?? to Cecil Spring Rice," August 15, 1917.
156 TNA, Foreign Office, FO 115/2236, "Taraknath Das to Emily Chadbourne," June 27, 1917.
157 *Ibid.*
158 TNA, Foreign Office, FO 115/2236, "Ellen N. La Motte to Taraknath Das," July 27, 1917.
159 In the letter, La Motte says that she intends to use a map, taken from "Millard's Eastern Question … showing spheres of influence" for a "first rate frontispiece"; see *ibid.* The map is taken from Thomas F. Millard, *Our Eastern Question: America's Contact with the Orient and the Trend of Relations with China and Japan* (New York: The Century Company, 1916), p. 381. It appears unattributed in *Peking Dust.*
160 TNA, Foreign Office, FO 115/2235, "N. to Major Thwaites," July 18, 1918.

161 Ruth Price, *The Lives of Agnes Smedley* (Oxford: Oxford University Press, 2005), p. 71.
162 TNA, Foreign Office, FO 115/2236, "Ellen N. La Motte to Taraknath Das," August 17, 1917.
163 NARA, Record Group 60: Records of the Department of Justice, "Post Wheeler to the Secretary of State," August 9, 1917.
164 Mukherjee, *Taraknath Das*, p. 147.
165 NARA, Record Group 60: Records of the Department of Justice, "Taraknath Das to Charles Recht," August 6, 1918.
166 NARA, Record Group 60: Records of the Department of Justice, Ellen N. La Motte, "The Case of Mrs. Emily C. Chadbourne and Ellen N. La Motte," May 14, 1919.
167 *Ibid.*
168 *Ibid.*
169 *Ibid.*
170 *Ibid.*
171 *Ibid.*
172 *Ibid.*
173 *Ibid.*
174 *Ibid.*
175 *Ibid.*
176 *Ibid.*
177 *Ibid.*
178 *Ibid.*
179 *Ibid.*
180 La Motte, *Drafts*, "The Spy."
181 *Ibid.*
182 *Ibid.*
183 *Ibid.*
184 *Ibid.*
185 *Ibid.*
186 AID, "La Motte to Alfred I. du Pont," August 1, 1918.
187 AID, "La Motte to Alfred I. du Pont," August 15, 1918.
188 In a letter from October 1954, La Motte's cousin, Jessie Ball du Pont, expressed her regret at the news of Sarre's death, and acknowledged how much she and Chadbourne would miss her friendship, suggesting the women maintained a relationship with Sarre until her death. See Jessie Ball du Pont Papers, Washington and Lee University, Lexington, VA, "Jessie Ball DuPont to Ellen N. La Motte," October 6, 1954.
189 See Harold Harris, Wendy E. Harris, and Diane Wiebe, *Yama Farms: A Most Unusual Catskills Resort* (Cragsmoor, NY: Cragsmoor Historical Society, 2006) for a general history of the inn.
190 AID, "La Motte to du Pont," December 4, 1918.

191 *Ibid.*

192 Judith Schwarz says the club started with twenty-five members who most likely met at Polly Halliday's restaurant, a gathering place for artists and bohemians in Greenwich Village. See Judith Schwarz, *Radical Feminists of Heterodoxy: Greenwich Village 1912–1940* (Norwich, VT: New Victoria Publishers, 1986), p. 17. Her book offers an excellent overview of the origins of the club and its evolution and membership. A contemporary source claims there were seventeen charter members; see "With the Members Sworn to Secrecy, Forty of New York's Prominent 'Advanced' Women Band into 'The Heterodoxy' and Meet to Eat and Decide Their Position on Problems of the Day," *New York Tribune* (November 24, 1914), p. 7.

193 Schwarz, *Radical Feminists*, p. 17.

194 *Ibid.*, p. 19.

195 See *ibid.*, pp. 7–16, for an overview of Howe's life.

196 IHIP, "Heterodoxy to Marie," 1920.

197 Cited in Schwarz, *Radical Feminists*, p. 17.

198 See JHMI, Ellen N. La Motte Collection, "Ellen N. La Motte to Amy Wesselhoeft von Erdberg," December 23, 1911, in which she says she sent her "Gilman's book," and in a later letter asks if Wesselhoeft von Erdberg is reading the *Forerunner* and comments that "Mrs. Gilman is so well worth while." See JHMI, Ellen N. La Motte Collection, "Ellen N. La Motte to Amy Wesselhoeft von Erdberg," March 20, 1912.

199 IHIP, "Inez Haynes Gillmore Irwin, War Diary, February 19, 1916–October 26, 1916."

200 *Ibid.*

201 *Ibid.*

202 *Ibid.*

203 Ellen N. La Motte, "Under Shell-Fire at Dunkirk," *Atlantic Monthly* (November 1915), p. 698.

204 IHIP, Irwin, War Diary. The Chicago Art Institute has works by Gauguin and Matisse that were donated by Chadbourne, and presumably Irwin saw them hanging in the Paris apartment in 1916. Chadbourne donated several thousand items to the Institute and La Motte a handful.

205 *Ibid.*

206 Their friendship was covered in the newspapers when Chadbourne was sued by her dressmaker, Beatrix F. Howard, for refusing to pay in full for a dress she had commissioned. As the story unraveled, Howard accused Koehler, "for many years … an intimate friend of Mrs. Chadbourne," of having "poisoned the mind of Mrs. Chadbourne against me." See "No Pay for Dress; Affinities Part," *Chicago Tribune* (June 6, 1907), p. 2. Chadbourne won the suit and Howard's business suffered a serious blow as a result of the bad publicity; see "Dresses Made in Chicago That Cost $6,000," *Chicago Tribune* (June 16, 1907), p. 39. In this same period of time, both Koehler

and Chadbourne received more negative coverage in the press when they were accused of smuggling: Koehler was accused of bringing undeclared jewels into the country–see "Girl Had Many Jewels," *New York Tribune* (March 7, 1907), p. 1–and Chadbourne, in a case on a much larger scale, of having tried to smuggle $80,000 worth of goods into the country on behalf of Isabella Stewart Gardner; see "Society Women Evade Customs; Fined $70,000," *Chicago Tribune* (August 19, 1908), p. 1.

207 The museum has the comb and pendant described by Irwin as well as a pearl necklace, all of which were donated by Chadbourne in 1952. It also has a filet necklace donated by Mrs. Alexander Tison in 1923. Tison's husband defended Koehler when she was accused of smuggling and Mrs. Tison, Anne Heyer Stevens, was a friend of Chadbourne's; presumably Chadbourne gave the necklace to Tison, who eventually donated it to the Met.

208 IHIP, Irwin, War Diary.

209 *Ibid.*

210 *Ibid.*

211 *Ibid.*

212 La Motte, *The Opium Monopoly*, p. xi.

213 *Ibid.*, p. xii.

214 *Ibid.*, p. xv.

215 *Ibid.*

216 *Ibid.*, p. xvi.

217 *Ibid.* p. 4.

218 *Ibid.*, pp. 21–22.

219 *Ibid.*, p. 73.

220 *Ibid.*

221 Ellen N. La Motte, *The Ethics of Opium* (New York: Century, 1924), p. 14.

222 *Ibid.*, p. 6.

223 AID, "Ellen N. La Motte to Alfred I. du Pont," November 5, 1920.

224 AID, "Ellen N. La Motte to Alfred I. du Pont," December 4, 1920.

225 GSABTP, "Ellen N. La Motte to Gertrude Stein," September 11, 1925.

226 "Whites in the Orient," *New York Times* (April 26, 1925), p. BR8.

227 MP, "Ellen N. La Motte to H. L. Mencken," May 15, 1924.

228 Private Collection, Ellen. N. La Motte, "The Psychology of Bobbing," unpublished.

229 Elinor Byrns was a lawyer in New York City and a member of Heterodoxy; perhaps she is the "Elinor" of the story.

230 La Motte, "The Psychology of Bobbing."

231 One person, Florence Crane, Jr., kept a diary as well, and it recounts her perspective as a seventeen-year-old traveling with her parents and governess. See Florence Crane, *Terrae Incognitae* (privately printed, 1927).

232 Private Collection, Ellen N. La Motte, "Egypt: Diary and Notes on a Trip Up the Nile, Cairo to Wadi Halfa, February and March, 1926"

(hereafter "Egypt: Diary and Notes"). For details concerning Prichard and Whittemore and their connection to Chadbourne and her art collecting, see R. S. Nelson, "The Art Collecting of Emily Crane Chadbourne and the Absence of Byzantine Art in Chicago," in C. Nielsen (ed.), *To Inspire and Instruct: A History of Medieval Art in Midwestern Museums* (Newcastle upon Tyne: Cambridge Scholars Publishing, 2008), pp. 131–148. D. M. Brodie, who arrived in Egypt with Cornelius Crane, was Crane's assistant; see N. E. Saul, *The Life and Times of Charles R. Crane, 1858–1939: American Businessman, Philanthropist, and a Founder of Russian Studies in America* (Lanham, MD: Lexington Books, 2013), p. 30.

233 La Motte, "Egypt: Diary and Notes," February 7, 1926.

234 GSABTP, "Emily Chadbourne to Gertrude Stein," February 24, 1926.

235 GSABTP, "Ellen N. La Motte to Gertrude Stein," June 12, 1926.

236 GSABTP, "Ellen N. La Motte to Gertrude Stein," February 13, 1929.

237 *Ibid.*

238 AID, "La Motte to du Pont," November 18, 1931.

Conclusion: The end of campaigning, 1930s–1961

When traveling on the Nile in 1926, La Motte watched "several Nubian children put off from the bank in little canoes … made of Standard Oil cans."[1] When the children followed the larger boats through the open locks, she observed to one of her traveling companions that "it is dangerous for that child to come in with these other boats … he'll be crushed to pieces in the lock" before recalling to herself, "Well, Citizen Fixit, this at least is not your responsibility!"[2] At this point she had been a crusader in the anti-tuberculosis, suffrage, and anti-opium campaigns for two decades. At times, her fatigue with being vigilant and outspoken in support of these causes made her want to retire from the constant struggle to improve the world around her. Ultimately, circumstances external to her would slow down her days of intense campaigning. The Great Depression curtailed her income and that of Emily Chadbourne, forcing them to return to the United States, where there was much less interest in the anti-opium campaign now that people had severe financial crises to contend with and conflict in Europe was increasing. As a result, her attention shifted in the last three decades of her life to focus on her burgeoning real-estate interests, financial investments, and circle of friends in Washington, DC and the Stone Ridge, NY area.

Before moving back to the United States in the fall of 1931, she and Chadbourne took their last major trip for some time and traveled to Abyssinia to see the coronation of Emperor Haile Selassie on November 2, 1930. Unfortunately, no letters or diary from her trip survive; instead, her article, published in *Harper's Magazine*, and unpublished draft manuscripts document her trip with "E." to "see … a great African spectacle."[3] She describes the journey from Marseilles to Djibouti on a "small, very old and dirty, and abominably crowded" boat and then the 500-mile train ride to the capital of Addis Ababa, where they stay in a converted "cow shed," the only accommodation thanks to the vast number of visitors in the city for the event.[4] The impetus for the piece seems to dispel the notion from her point of view that "this bit of Africa, the only bit not under European control, was progressive and up-to-date, with an active, enlightened ruler, making great strides to keep up his Western neighbors."[5] To buttress her view, she focuses on what she sees as poor living conditions, "mud huts ... covered with thatch" and a dearth of "arts and crafts or handiwork of any kind. The Abyssinians are too poor and too primitive, with their lives as bare of refinement as any other African peoples."[6] The article continues in this vein, offering critiques of the food and water quality and sharing concerns about disease. She also highlights the hypocrisy of the enormous expense of the coronation and the fact that most of the money was spent abroad acquiring "resplendent uniforms, costly wines, foreign food, lion-skin busbys made in England, furniture, coaches, horses."[7] Despite having traveled long and far to reach the coronation, La Motte could find nothing redemptive in the experience.

She was certainly painted as sober and bitter in Evelyn Waugh's short portrait of her and Chadbourne, in which he describes them as "two formidable ladies in knitted suits and topis; though unrelated by blood, long companionship had made them almost indistinguishable, square-jawed, tight-lipped, with hard, discontented eyes. For them the whole coronation was a profound disappointment .... They were out for Vice. They were collecting material, in fact, for a little book on the subject .... Prostitution and drug traffic comprised their modest interests, and they were too dense to find evidence of either."[8] His vision of them is as bleak and prejudiced as La Motte's of Ethiopia. In Waugh's vision the two women are unhappy spinster-types devoid of humor and intelligence and reduced to caricatures of female reformers.

In La Motte's vision the people of Ethiopia are similarly devoid of individual characteristics, as she can see them only through the prism of poverty and illness. La Motte's racism was most virulent in relation to black people, whether African Americans or Africans, undoubtedly a reflection of the racist environment in which she was raised and her family's and friends' assumptions regarding white superiority. Her cousin and frequent correspondent, Alfred I. du Pont, for example, referred to African Americans as "chocolate drops."[9] Chadbourne, in a letter to Gertrude Stein praising a performance of her opera, *Four Saints in Three Acts*, opined that she had "never before cared for negroes,"[10] and La Motte had already told Stein years earlier that a student from Yale had written asking to meet with her to discuss opium and that she and Chadbourne had "got into panic fear lest he be a negro," then amended her comments, saying "I wouldn't mind myself, but Em has her prejudices," a statement that seems to directly contradict the "panic fear" she confessed to experiencing at the very idea that an African American student might visit her home.[11]

This racism, evident as early as her tuberculosis writings from 1905 to 1913 and her "humorous" sketches of her African American patients, is difficult to reconcile with some of her advocacy work, in which she pointed to the structural injustices endured by women and African Americans and campaigned on behalf of colonized people subject to corrupt policies that facilitated the sale of drugs to them while barring their sale in European countries populated primarily by whites. She understood the hypocrisy of allowing for these kinds of practices so that countries like Great Britain could fill their coffers while sacrificing the bodies and minds of people of color. Yet, like many other progressives, she shared racist views that colored her understanding of the world she was trying to improve and assumed white superiority was a given. She lived to see the start of the Civil Rights movement, but there is no documentation of whether she embraced the structural changes activists were demanding in order to create a more just society.

Once they settled into living in the United States again, she and Chadbourne took up residence at 2000 Massachusetts Avenue, the Blaine Mansion on Dupont Circle that was converted from a single-family home into "a high-end apartment house."[12] They had been using it as a base since at least 1925, when they would stay there on one of their many visits from London to Washington, DC. However, in May 1932, no longer receiving dividends from the Crane Company, Chadbourne had to give it up; the two women became "interested in the economies of the Piggly Wiggly," most likely the first time in her life that Emily Chadbourne had ever had to think about how to save money on groceries and to be involved in purchasing them, and made Sally Tock's in Stone Ridge their primary residence.[13] Chadbourne had purchased the house in Stone Ridge after the end of World War One and kept it until her death. She spent part of every year there, even opening a cosmetics business that operated from her home for a time in the 1930s,[14] and La Motte often joined her for extended stays; they became part of the local community, with La Motte giving talks when she was still involved in the anti-opium campaign in the 1920s and 1930s and Chadbourne becoming active in supporting the arts in the area, including the Senate House in nearby Kingston.[15]

When in Washington, La Motte took an interest in the reason for their straitened circumstances, the stock market crash, and attended hearings conducted by the Senate Banking and Finance Committee that were part of the investigation into the buying and selling of stocks and securities. She explained to her cousin that the hearings were "packed, more women than men, and every one feverishly anxious to find out how they have been swindled."[16] Her own finances would have been in dire straits had her cousin not set up a trust for her, for which, she wrote to him, "every day I am more grateful to you for all you have done for me, and for that trust money … [in] these hard times, I don't know what I should do without this constant and generous check … I can never thank you enough."[17]

She had more time to attend hearings, given that her publishing career was on the wane: after her move to Washington, DC in the fall of 1931, she published two more articles on opium and completed research at the Library of Congress for the Field Museum for material to be on exhibit at the 1933 Chicago's World Fair, a "grand chance to show up the opium trade!"[18] In a complete change of pace she also published an article, "Miniature Fireplaces," in *Antiques* magazine. The article describes her collection of miniature fireplaces and her pleasure in collecting and restoring these items.[19] In an unexpected turn, her censored 1916 book of sketches of nursing on the Western Front during World War One, *The Backwash of War*, was republished with the addition of a new story, "Esmeralda." According to a letter she wrote to her cousin, Putnam's wanted to add two stories, which she gave to them, but in the end added only the one, written in 1917.[20] The book was issued by Putnam's with a dust jacket that proclaimed it was "as overwhelming as parts of *All Quiet on the Western Front*," "as

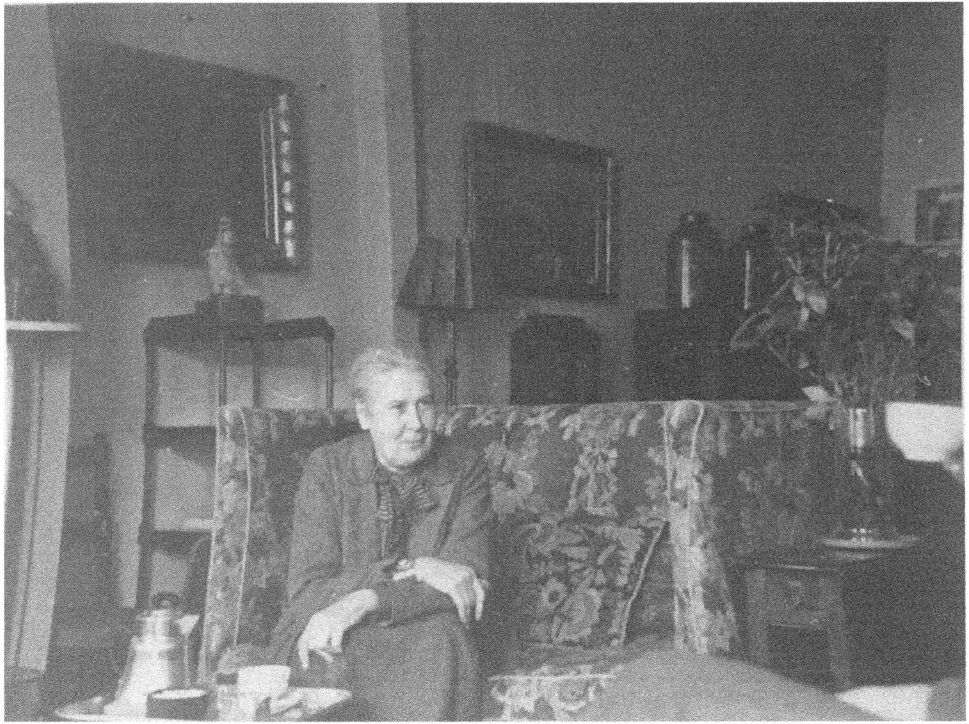

Figure 15 Portrait of La Motte, undated

moving as parts of *A Farewell to Arms*," and possessed "the accuracy and simplicity encountered only in such truly great books as *The Red Badge of Courage*."[21] La Motte must have reveled in comparisons to novels such as those by Remarque and Hemingway that had emerged as fundamental texts in the canon of literature of World War One. Reviewers drew similar comparisons with those writers plus Dos Passos and made the point that the book "will cause no sensation," despite its depiction of the ugly side of war, "because the public mind is several jumps ahead of the author in expectations of greater dreadfulness in the next war."[22] For once, La Motte was unable to shock her audiences and would not incur the kind of criticism lodged against *The Backwash of War* in 1916; what was seen as too grim then now matched current disillusioned understandings of past and future wars. She was probably less thrilled that the inside of the dust jacket dramatically declared that "the author, who was a nurse, has written nothing since."[23] In fact, La Motte's most productive writing period would come after the war, when she found her passion and voice in the anti-opium campaign.

In the 1930s, recognition for her opium work culminated in her being awarded the Lin Tse Hsu Memorial Medal in a ceremony at the Chinese Legation in Washington, DC, on February 9, 1930, alongside three other recipients, Stephen G. Porter, Republican representative for Pennsylvania; Mrs. Elizabeth Wright; and Dr. W. W. Willoughby, a political science professor at Johns Hopkins University. The ceremony commemorated the ninetieth anniversary of the destruction of a million dollars' worth of opium by the Chinese and newspaper coverage acknowledged La Motte as "an international authority on combating drug traffic."[24] This recognition is surely why she was invited to the White House in December 1933, her second of at least three invitations, although in a letter to her cousin she said she "had no idea why" she had been invited, even though she had gone "to see Mrs. Roosevelt a couple of times, about opium."[25] Despite being in close proximity to the political power of Washington, DC she was unable to leverage the contacts she did have to continue a vigorous fight against opium, and at the end of June 1935, supported with a check given to her after her cousin's death at the end of April of that year, she returned to Europe with Chadbourne and her sister-in-law, Florence Crane, married to Chadbourne's brother, Richard Crane,

Jr. Their intention was to go to London, then La Motte would continue on to Geneva to "catch up with the opium at first hand."[26] Her plans, however, did not materialize, because the League of Nations Opium Committee would not be meeting until November and it was too expensive to make the trip.[27] La Motte wrote more frankly from England to Gertrude Stein to explain they could not "afford" the trip over, having recently realized how much money they were losing because of the exchange rates. She also added that although she was enjoying being back and seeing friends, she "could never live [t]here again. It is funny how you completely finish with a thing."[28] As far as the record shows, after almost two decades of living and traveling in Europe, this may have been her last trip to the place that had served as her second home and played such a pivotal role in fostering her artistic, intellectual, and activist aspirations.

Europe came to her, however, in the form of Gertrude Stein and Alice B. Toklas when the two women embarked on their legendary six-month tour of America in the fall of 1934. La Motte and Chadbourne had kept up a steady if occasional correspondence with Stein and Toklas over the years before *The Autobiography of Alice B. Toklas* was published in 1933, and its appearance prompted La Motte to write to Stein that "we are both crazy over your autobiography, and our social standing has gone up tremendously, through having been mentioned in it."[29] By the end of October Chadbourne and La Motte were writing to Stein to make preliminary plans to meet in Baltimore. La Motte later wrote to Toklas to plan Stein's visit to the Washington, DC area, including helping to orchestrate an invitation to have tea with Eleanor Roosevelt.[30] No doubt their social standing was further bolstered when Stein's *Everybody's Autobiography* was published in 1937 and acknowledged La Motte, who spent New Year's Eve with Stein in Virginia and then drove her "through the rest of Virginia."[31]

Stein and Toklas' trip brought the internationalism La Motte had once enjoyed to her; otherwise, La Motte's international travel in the 1930s was limited: she took a trip to Panama in in 1934 to help Chadbourne, who was attending to her niece's husband, William Albert Robinson, who had had an attack of appendicitis and would require weeks of recovery; La Motte was very excited to see "the American Tropics," her sense of adventure fully engaged as she made hasty preparations to load her "Chev" on the boat to the canal zone.[32] Travel like this excited and stimulated her, and as she aged, it was a way of testing her capacity to adapt to new circumstances; she proudly reported to her cousin that, having quickly learned to drive on the left-hand side, she felt satisfied that she still had "a flexible and adjustable mind."[33]

Curtailed by finances and eventually the effects of age, these kinds of trips ended and she spent her time physically in the United States, although she joined the Society of Woman Geographers in 1931, allowing her to enjoy socializing with women who shared her interests in travel and politics. Her notes for their annual bulletin, which she completed through 1960, show her activities declining in the mid to late 1930s, although as late as 1944 she said she had "several articles on opium accepted, but not yet published"[34]–these do not seem to have to have materialized in print–until she became "professionally inactive."[35]

She reported to the Society of Woman Geographers in 1942 that "for the past several years I have been buying old Georgetown houses and restoring or remodeling them–and them selling them. … As a Geographer don't you think I am a little weak? Am I really eligible?"[36] While the buying and selling of real estate certainly did not fall into the categories of activities that got women invited into the Society, it became a replacement for the excitement of travel and adventure that La Motte used to enjoy prior to the 1930s. She began buying houses in the Georgetown area of Washington, DC in the late 1930s as a way to make money and to use her interest in and dexterity with financial investments. It was a risky enterprise during economic hard times and the difficulty of selling–one house was on the market for a year–put her in "a state of jitters."[37] Despite her anxieties about the prospect of finding buyers, she bought another house two years later on credit that she hoped to turn around and sell at a profit.[38] She was more optimistic and found the interest in the house to be "very exciting" due to the "booming" real-estate market in Washington.[39] She would continue to buy and sell houses into the 1940s, staying busy with the transactions helped to distract her from "the war."[40] Ever the pioneer, La Motte was the first woman to be allowed into the Georgetown Citizens' Association in 1945 after the group lifted a ban on female membership earlier that year.[41] She stayed deeply connected to the neighborhood until her death, when she owned two houses in the area.

Her knowledge of historic homes and familiarity with the suffrage movement undoubtedly made her a logical choice to chair the House Committee of the National Woman's Party by Florence Bayard Hilles. Hilles was an old friend and came from the Bayard family of Delaware, who had close ties to the du Ponts. La Motte and her cousin occasionally referred to Hilles or her sister, Louise Lee Angell, in their letters, with La Motte having more contact with Hilles and her cousin with Angell, whom he saw as having a "pretty rough row to hoe."[42] La Motte in turn shared a few tidbits about seeing Hilles in London for a week, "this first real visit … in years, and we both enjoyed it so much."[43] The women kept up their friendship after La Motte returned to live in the United States and Hilles asked her in 1938 to help with the work of restoring one of the houses adjoining the headquarters of the Party–what is today the Belmont-Paul Women's Equality National Monument–and La Motte wrote that she was "idiot enough to accept" this work that had been keeping her busy since November.[44] Eight months later, she reported that she was still having "a hectic time with the National Woman's Party," which she "inadvertently got mixed up with–largely through Florence Bayard. We had three prolonged meetings yesterday and when they finish up with all their meetings (this is their big annual one) I hope to make my escape. And once escaped–never again!"[45] She fulfilled her obligations to complete the project, which included restoring the smaller building then "mov[ing] all the offices into it from the big house" so that they could "let all those handsome rooms in the main house at good rate, to carry the expense."[46] Like so much of her work, this too was controversial, and she commented, "it has taken a lot of time and thought and the House Committee is getting pretty unpopular."[47] She distances herself from the Party in these comments, but she appears in several photographs documenting the incorporation of the World Woman's Party, taken in 1938, suggesting she may have been more involved than her letters suggest.[48] Nonetheless, it appears that after the restoration project was complete, no longer feeling the ardor she used to have for the suffrage cause, she distanced herself from the Party and their work.

La Motte's life in the 1940s–1950s remained split between her real-estate interests and assisting Chadbourne with her affairs. La Motte did her taxes for her, something that must have been a significant undertaking given her assets,[49] helped her sort out her estate,[50] and oversaw work done on several of her houses.[51] This role as financial manager clearly made Chadbourne's family uneasy, presumably in large part because she was a woman managing her partner's affairs. Chadbourne's niece, Margaret C.-L. Gildea, fifteen years after her aunt's death, left an account in which she observed that La Motte was Chadbourne's "closest and most intimate friend," who "handle[d] her financial affairs."[52] She edges toward dismissing La Motte as being from "the poor branch of the LaMotte DuPont family," who received financial advice from Alfred I. du Pont.[53] By 1940, du Pont had been dead five years and La Motte was making decisions based on her research and business acumen, and Gildea had to admit grudgingly that La Motte "made over $1,000,000 for her."[54] The source of Gildea's bitterness was that La Motte's actions resulted in Chadbourne's giving control of the Crane Company, via proxy, to a businessman who had been attempting to take over the faltering company. This action ultimately saved the company even as it meant that it passed out of family hands, something Chadbourne's father had forbidden his descendants from permitting. Her father had been dead many years at this point and the company was facing unforeseen challenges in the post-World War Two environment; it was a good move to hand over control even if it defied the patriarchal authority of its founder, something Gildea in her account invests in, placing blame on La Motte for violating this paternal edict. Never one to defer to male authority or to bow to sentimentality, La Motte understood the benefits of allowing someone new to take control, and even Gildea had to admit that the company began to do "much better" and those holding stock, herself included, "prospered."[55]

Gildea also provides the only account of the end of both women's lives, although in reference to La Motte's death, she can say only that her aunt was "desolated" at the loss of her friend.[56] La Motte's last known surviving letter dates from December 1959 and is full of typos, a sign of her failing eyesight, but in it she still displays a keen sense of humor and assures her correspondent that she is "tough as an [old] hickory nut" and takes a walk to see Chadbourne every morning, though she needed to do so with assistance.[57] Fifteen months later, on March 2, 1961, she died at home in Washington, DC and was buried in Oak

Hill Cemetery in the Georgetown area. Her grave is simply marked with her name and birth and death dates. She is not surrounded by the graves of her family members; rather, her final resting place is as independent as the way she lived her life: she is on her own in a place that she made into her intellectual and personal home.

La Motte would probably have been pleased with the newspaper coverage of her death. Papers in Wilmington and Baltimore ran obituaries in recognition of her connection to those cities, as did the *New York Times*. Its obituary is titled, "Ellen La Motte, Author, Was 87,"[58] an attribution that she would have particularly enjoyed. She began her professional life as a highly trained nurse, and nursing readied her to write and speak well, to take and defend controversial positions, and to consider the relationship between the patient's rights and wellbeing and the welfare of the larger community. She used that knowledge as she experienced the consequences of the first world-wide modern war and the fallout of colonialism and exploitation in the opium trade. Her goal in 1898 when she was a twenty-five-year-old woman who had never had any kind of job was, according to Georgina Caird Ross, her interviewer, to "make something out of her life."[59] Sixty-three years later, La Motte could boast of a career that spanned four decades and included seven books and dozens of articles about topics as diverse as nursing, tuberculosis, suffrage, World War One, and opium, and that she had firmly established herself as a nurse, writer, and activist.

Notes

1 La Motte, "Egypt: Diary and Notes."
2 *Ibid.*
3 Ellen, N. La Motte, "A Coronation in Abyssinia," *Harper's Magazine* (April 1931), pp. 574–584.
4 *Ibid.*, p. 575.
5 *Ibid.*, p. 576.
6 *Ibid.*
7 *Ibid.*, p. 581.
8 Evelyn Waugh, *Remote People* (London: Penguin Books, 2002), p. 34.
9 AID, "Alfred I. du Pont to Ellen N. La Motte," March 30, 1922.
10 GSABTP, "Emily Chadbourne to Gertrude Stein," February 14, 1932.
11 GSABTP, "La Motte to Stein," August 7, 1925.

12 Stephen A. Hansen, "What Once Was: The Blaine Mansion at Dupont Circle," *InTowner* (Washington, DC) (November 11, 2013). The article provides background on the creation of the mansion, which is still standing.
13 AID, "Ellen N. La Motte to Alfred I du Pont," May 17, 1932.
14 "Cosmetics Firm Is Incorporated," *Kingston Daily Freeman* (April 2, 1937), p. 2.
15 "Mrs. Emily Chadbourne Dies, Aided Senate House, Museum," *Kingston Daily Freeman* (December 24, 1964), p. 1.
16 AID, "La Motte to du Pont," April 27, 1932.
17 AID, "La Motte to du Pont," April 13, 1932.
18 JBDP, "Ellen N. La Motte to Jessie Ball du Pont," November 17, 1932.
19 Ellen N. La Motte, "Miniature Fireplaces," *Antiques* (June 1932), pp. 272–274.
20 AID, "La Motte to du Pont," June 30, 1934. See Chapter 4 for a discussion of the genesis of "Esmeralda."
21 Ellen N. La Motte, *The Backwash of War* (New York: G. P. Putnam's Sons, 1934), dust jacket.
22 George Currie, "Passed in Review," *Brooklyn Daily Eagle* (August 25, 1934), p. 16.
23 La Motte, *The Backwash of War*, dust jacket.
24 "Wilmington Woman Honored by China," *Wilmington Star* (March 2, 1930).
25 AID, "La Motte to du Pont," January 7, 1934.
26 JBDP, "La Motte to Ball du Pont," June 9, 1935.
27 JBDP, "La Motte to Ball du Pont," August 30, 1935.
28 GSABTP, "La Motte to Gertrude Stein," July 14, 1935.
29 GSABTP, "Chadbourne to Stein," February 14, 1934. La Motte added a postscript to Chadbourne's letter to Stein.
30 GSABTP, "Ellen N. La Motte to Alice B. Toklas," December 20, 1934.
31 Gertrude Stein, *Everybody's Autobiography* (New York: Cooper Square Publishers, 1971), 235.
32 AID, "La Motte to du Pont," June 5, 1934.
33 AID, "La Motte to du Pont," June 30, 1934.
34 Ellen Newbold La Motte, "For the 1945 Bulletin of the Society of Woman Geographers," I:19, Society of Woman Geographers Records (hereafter SWGR), Manuscript Division, Library of Congress, Washington, DC.
35 La Motte, "For the 1951 Bulletin of the Society of Woman Geographers," SWGR.
36 La Motte, "For the 1942 Bulletin of the Society of Woman Geographers," SWGR.
37 JBDP, "La Motte to Ball du Pont," May 10, 1938.
38 JBDP, "La Motte to Ball du Pont, September 10, 1940.
39 *Ibid.*
40 JBDP, "La Motte to Ball du Pont," May 4, 1943.
41 "Georgetown Group Breaks Precedent, Admits Women," *Evening Star* (Washington, DC) (November 27, 1945), p. A-9.
42 AID, "Du Pont to La Motte," November 17, 1919.

43 AID, "La Motte to du Pont," May 22, 1931.
44 JBDP, "La Motte to Ball du Pont," March 20, 1939.
45 JBDP, "La Motte to Ball du Pont," November 18, 1939.
46 JBDP, "La Motte to Ball du Pont," March 20, 1939.
47 *Ibid.*
48 Papers of Alice Paul, 1785–1985, Schlesinger Library, Radcliffe Institute, Harvard University, Cambridge, MA, "Photographs of Officers and World Woman's Party Headquarters, Geneva, Switzerland, n.d."
49 JBDP, "La Motte to Ball du Pont," January 23, 1947.
50 JBDP, "La Motte to Ball du Pont," January 31, 1947.
51 JBDP, "La Motte to Ball du Pont," October 20, 1947.
52 CHM, Crane Family and Lillie Family Papers, 1833–1978 (bulk 1890s–1960s), "Essay by Margaret Crane Lillie Gildea Discussing Crane Family Relations with the Crane Company, with Emphasis on Emily Crane Chadbourne (1871–1964), Written 1978," p. 1.
53 *Ibid.*
54 *Ibid.*
55 *Ibid.*, p. 19.
56 *Ibid.*
57 JBDP, "La Motte to Ball du Pont," October 1, 1959.
58 "Ellen La Motte, Author, Was 87," *New York Times* (March 4, 1961), p. 23.
59 Georgina Caird Ross, JHMI, Student Applications, "Notes from Interview with Ellen La Motte," July 19, 1898.

Index

Note: page references in *italic* refer to figures.

EU authorised representative for GPSR:
Easy Access System Europe, Mustamäe tee 50,
10621 Tallinn, Estonia
gpsr.requests@easproject.com

www.ingramcontent.com/pod-product-compliance
Ingram Content Group UK Ltd.
Pitfield, Milton Keynes, MK11 3LW, UK
UKHW021833100926
8556IPUK00004B/323
* 9 7 8 1 5 2 6 1 2 9 5 1 2 *